High-Protein, Low-Carb, Low-Sugar

COOKBOOK

Lose Up to 20 Pounds in 3 Months with 120g Protein, 1200-1600 Calories a day and low carb Recipes (Sample Meal Plans and 3-Month Planner Included)

Avery Stoneheart

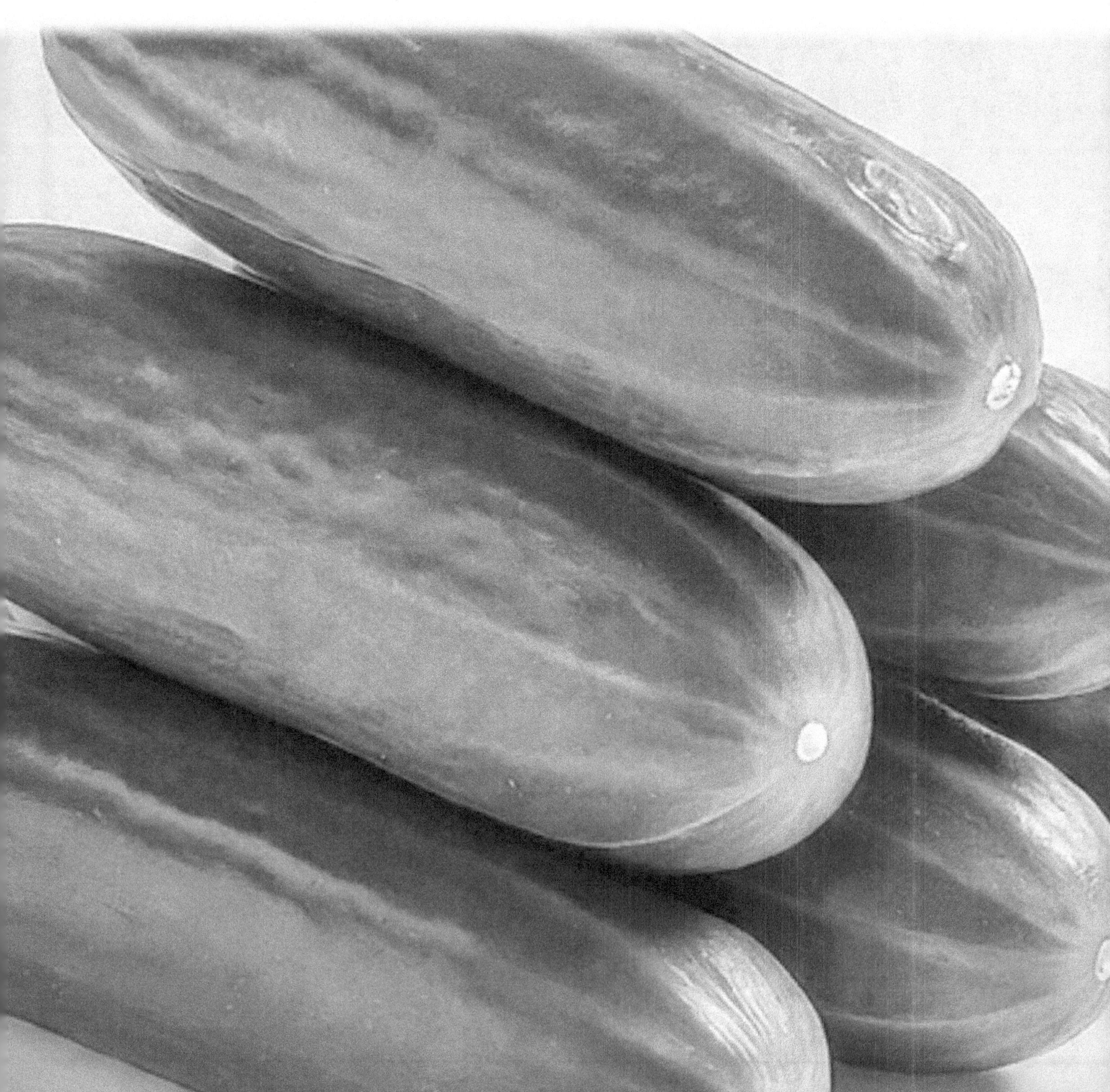

TABLE OF CONENTS

INTRODUCTION

My Story

I haven't always been the picture of health. I struggled with my own weight for years, the emotional rollercoaster of quick-fix diets leaving me feeling defeated. But that struggle ignited a fire in me. I immersed myself in nutrition, determined to find a way out of the fog of fad diets and misinformation. It was a journey of scientific discovery, of trial and error, and most importantly, of seeing the incredible transformations of my clients.

People just like you, tired of the weight loss struggle, who walked through my door feeling hopeless. Together, we embarked on a journey – not about deprivation, but about fueling their bodies for success. I witnessed firsthand the power of a high-protein, low-carb, and low-sugar approach. It wasn't magic, it was science.

The Science

Let's be real – our bodies are designed to thrive on real, whole foods. When we flood them with sugar and processed carbs, chaos happens. Our blood sugar spikes and crashes, hormones get out of whack, and we store fat instead of burning it. But, when we give our bodies high-quality protein, the building blocks of our cells, it's a game-changer. Protein keeps you feeling full, boosts your metabolism, and helps you preserve precious muscle mass when you're in a calorie deficit. Cutting back on those sneaky sugars and refined carbs? That's where we unlock stable energy, better sleep, and say goodbye to those relentless cravings.

Consistency is Queen (or King!)

This isn't a get-slim-quick scheme. This is a lifestyle shift. It's about creating habits and finding a way of eating that makes you feel energized and empowered. Will there be challenges? Absolutely! But that's where I come in. I'll be your biggest cheerleader, the accountability you crave, and the nutrition guru in your corner. Step by step, you'll gain the knowledge and skills to reach your goals… and this time, keep them off for good.

Are you ready to ditch the diet mentality and embrace a sustainable path to the body you deserve? Let's do this!

Chapter 1: The Foundations

Macronutrients: Your Body's Building Blocks

Think of food as more than just calories. The things we eat are made up of three key players: proteins, carbohydrates, and fats. These are called macronutrients – "macro" because our bodies need them in relatively large amounts. Each one plays a vital role in keeping us healthy, but also directly affects our weight loss journey.

Protein: The Hunger-Busting Superhero

- **What it is:** Think of protein as the building blocks of your body. It makes up your muscles, organs, skin, hair – even your hormones and enzymes.
- **Sources:** Chicken, fish, lean meat, eggs, beans, lentils, Greek yogurt, nuts, seeds.
- **Weight Loss Power:** Protein is the most satiating of all the macros, meaning it keeps you feeling full for longer. It also helps preserve muscle mass when you're losing weight, which boosts your metabolism and makes it easier to maintain your results.

Carbohydrates: Fuel With a Caveat

- **What they are:** Carbs are your body's primary energy source. They come in different forms:
    - Simple carbs: Sugars (found in candy, processed foods, even fruit), easily broken down for quick energy.
    - Complex carbs: Starches and fiber (found in whole grains, vegetables, beans), take longer to digest, providing sustained energy.
- **Sources:** Bread, pasta, rice, fruits, vegetables, sugary drinks, desserts.
- **Weight Loss Power:** Simple carbs can lead to blood sugar spikes and crashes, leaving you hungry and prone to overeating. Complex carbs are a better bet, especially fiber-rich ones that support healthy digestion and keep you full.

Fats: Not the Enemy

- **What they are:** Fats are essential for absorbing vitamins, protecting organs, and keeping our cell membranes healthy.
- **Sources:** Healthy fats include nuts, seeds, avocado, olive oil, fatty fish. Unhealthy fats include deep-fried foods, processed meats, and highly processed oils.
- **Weight Loss Power:** Fats are calorie-dense, so moderation is key. But healthy fats help with satiety and contribute to a balanced, sustainable diet.

It's not about eliminating any single macronutrient. It's about finding the right balance for your unique needs and goals. This high-protein, low-carb, and low-sugar approach prioritizes protein and healthy fats for maximizing fullness and minimizing those blood sugar rollercoasters.

Unlocking Your Personal Calorie & Protein Code

Forget one-size-fits-all diets! To see real results, we need to tailor your plan. Think of this as cracking a code – figuring out just how much fuel your body needs to shed pounds while still feeling fueled and energized. Here's how we'll do it:

<u>Step 1: Finding Your Calorie Target</u>

We'll start by calculating your Basal Metabolic Rate (BMR). This is the number of calories your body burns simply by existing. You can use a reliable online calculator like the one on Calculator.net (https://www.calculator.net/bmr-calculator.html). Don't worry, it's easy to use! Then, we'll factor in your activity level. More active? You'll need a few extra calories to fuel those workouts. This gives us your total daily calorie target. To target weight loss, we'll aim for a modest calorie deficit – burning a bit more than you take in.

<u>Step 2: The Protein Power-Up</u>

Remember, this plan is all about protein! It's your secret weapon against hunger and muscle loss. We'll aim for a good chunk of your daily calories to come from protein sources. I'll provide a simple formula that takes your body weight into account – giving you a personalized protein goal in grams.

The Fine-Tuning

These calculations get us super close. But listen, your body is unique! We'll adjust as we go based on how *you* feel and how the scale is moving. This isn't about getting it perfect on day one, it's about making progress and finding what works best for you long-term.

Busting a Common Myth: Starvation Mode

You might have heard horror stories – if you eat too few calories, your body panics and holds onto weight. It's true that drastic calorie cutting can backfire. That's why we're doing this thoughtfully. A modest calorie deficit and plenty of protein will prevent the dreaded "starvation mode" and keep you on the path to success.

What You'll Need:

- A calculator (or you can use an online BMR calculator)
- Your height and weight
- A basic understanding of your daily activity level (sedentary, moderately active, etc.)

Let's Do Some Math!

Meet Alex (Male)

Alex is a 35-year-old man who's 5'10" tall and weighs 185 pounds. He has a desk job but tries to hit the gym 3-4 times a week. His goal is to lose weight, build some muscle, and feel more energized.

Step 1: Calculating Alex's BMR

We'll use a common formula like the Mifflin-St Jeor equation. There are different ones out there, and we can choose the most appropriate one together! Just to illustrate:

- Men: BMR = (10 x weight in kg) + (6.25 x height in cm) - (5 x age) + 5

Let's convert Alex's measurements:

- Weight: 185 pounds = 83.9 kg
- Height: 5'10" = 177.8 cm

Plugging it in: (10 x 83.9) + (6.25 x 177.8) - (5 x 35) + 5 = 1865 calories

This means Alex's body burns about 1865 calories per day just by existing.

Step 2: Activity Factor

Since Alex is moderately active, we'll multiply his BMR by 1.55. This gives us around 2890 calories as his maintenance level (the amount where he'd neither gain nor lose weight).

To create a calorie deficit for weight loss, we'll subtract around 300-500 calories from that number. Let's aim for a target of 2500 calories per day.

<u>**Step 3: Protein Power**</u>

Since Alex wants to build muscle, we might recommend a slightly higher protein intake, around 1.2-1.5 grams per pound of bodyweight.

- 185 pounds x 1.2 gram/pound = 222 grams protein per day (minimum)
- 185 pounds x 1.5 grams/pound = 277 grams protein per day (maximum)

We could suggest Alex starts around the middle of that range, maybe 250 grams of protein a day.

The Fine-Tuning

We'll tell Alex to track his food intake, strength training progress, energy levels, and weight loss for a couple of weeks. If he's not seeing results or feels constantly hungry, we might tweak his calorie or protein targets slightly.

Meet Olivia(Female)

Olivia is a 35-year-old woman who's 5'6" tall and weighs 160 pounds. She has a desk job but tries to hit the gym 3-4 times a week. Her goal is to lose weight and feel more energized.

<u>**Step 1: Calculating Olivia's BMR**</u>

We'll use a common formula like the Mifflin-St Jeor equation. There are different ones out there, and we can choose the most appropriate one together! Just to illustrate:

- Women: BMR = (10 x weight in kg) + (6.25 x height in cm) - (5 x age) - 161

Let's convert Olivia's measurements:

- Weight: 160 pounds = 72.6 kg
- Height: 5'6" = 167.6 cm

Plugging it in: (10 x 72.6) + (6.25 x 167.6) - (5 x 35) - 161 = 1460 calories

This means Olivia's body burns about 1460 calories per day just by existing.

<u>**Step 2: Activity Factor**</u>

Since Olivia is moderately active, we'll multiply her BMR by 1.55. This gives us around 2263 calories as her maintenance level (the amount where she'd neither gain nor lose weight).

To create a calorie deficit for weight loss, we'll subtract around 300-500 calories from that number. Let's aim for a target of 1800 calories per day.

<u>**Step 3: Protein Power**</u>

On a high-protein plan, a good baseline is around 1 gram of protein per pound of bodyweight. For Olivia:

- 160 pounds x 1 gram/pound = 160 grams of protein per day.

The Fine-Tuning

We'll tell Olivia to track her food intake, energy levels, and weight loss progress for a couple of weeks. If she's not seeing results or feels constantly hungry, we might tweak her calorie or protein targets slightly.

Chapter 2: Stocking Your Kitchen for Success

Think of your kitchen as your weight loss headquarters! Stocking it with the right ingredients sets you up to easily whip up tasty, satisfying meals that align with your high-protein, low-carb, and low-sugar plan. Let's break it down:

The Ultimate Shopping List

We'll focus on fresh, whole foods with long-lasting staples to round things out. Here's your go-to guide:

Proteins:

- ✓ Chicken breast, turkey breast, lean beef, fish (salmon, tuna, cod, etc.)
- ✓ Shellfish (shrimp, scallops, etc.)
- ✓ Eggs
- ✓ Greek yogurt, cottage cheese
- ✓ Lentils, beans (kidney, black, etc.)

Veggies:

- ✓ Leafy greens: Spinach, kale, lettuce
- ✓ Cruciferous veggies: Broccoli, cauliflower, Brussels sprouts
- ✓ Other favorites: Bell peppers, zucchini, tomatoes, cucumbers, mushrooms

Healthy Fats:

- ✓ Avocados
- ✓ Olive oil
- ✓ Nuts (almonds, walnuts, etc.) and seeds (pumpkin, sunflower)
- ✓ Nut butters (peanut, almond) – unsweetened, if possible

Fruits:

- ✓ Stick to lower-sugar options like berries (blueberries, raspberries, strawberries)

Pantry Staples

These are your backup crew, helping you pull together a meal in a pinch:

- Canned tuna or salmon
- Canned beans (rinse well to reduce sodium)
- Pre-cooked lentils
- Quinoa
- Whole-grain or Ezekiel bread
- Oats
- Protein powder (look for low-sugar options)

Spice Up Your Life!

Flavor is your BFF on this plan! A well-stocked spice rack means no more boring meals. Essentials include:

- Salt, black pepper, garlic powder, onion powder, paprika, cumin, chili powder
- Italian seasoning, dried herbs (basil, oregano, thyme)
- Fresh herbs when possible (cilantro, parsley)
- Hot sauce, mustard, low-sugar salsa, vinegars

Recipe Tie-Ins

- **Remember that "Tuna Power Salad" from Chapter 4?** Make sure you always have canned tuna and greens on hand!
- **Craving those "Spicy Lentil & Chicken Soup" vibes?** Keep canned tomatoes, lentils, and spices stocked.
- **Love the "Cottage Cheese Delight?"** Don't let those berries run out!

Smart Shopping Tips

- **Plan Ahead:** A meal plan means no impulse buys that derail your goals.
- **Hit the Perimeter:** That's where most of the whole foods live.
- **Read Labels:** Look for simple ingredient lists, and watch those added sugars!

Chapter 3: Meal Planning for Weight Loss Success

We've got your kitchen stocked, now let's turn those ingredients into satisfying and balanced meals! This isn't about deprivation; it's about finding what works for you, keeping it simple, and setting yourself up for long-term success.

Building Balanced Meals

Think of each meal like a puzzle with three key pieces:

1. **The Protein Powerhouse:** Aim for a good palm-sized portion of your chosen protein – a chicken breast, a few ounces of fish, a scoop of lentils, etc. This is your hunger-buster and muscle preserver.
2. **The Veggie Volume:** Fill half your plate with colorful veggies. Think greens, broccoli, peppers, you name it! They add fiber for fullness, plus vitamins and minerals for overall health.
3. **Healthy Fats for Flavor:** A drizzle of olive oil, a sprinkle of nuts, a dollop of avocado. Fats slow digestion for lasting energy and help you absorb those veggie nutrients.

Recipe Tie-Ins

- **"Greek Yogurt Marinated Chicken" + a big salad + olive oil dressing?** Perfect!
- **Lentil soup + a side of roasted veggies?** Super satisfying combo.
- **Tuna steak over quinoa + steamed broccoli?** Easy and balanced.

Portion Pointers

No need to count calories meticulously! Use visual cues:

- Protein: Palm-sized portion
- Veggies: Take up half your plate
- Healthy Fats: A thumb-sized amount per meal

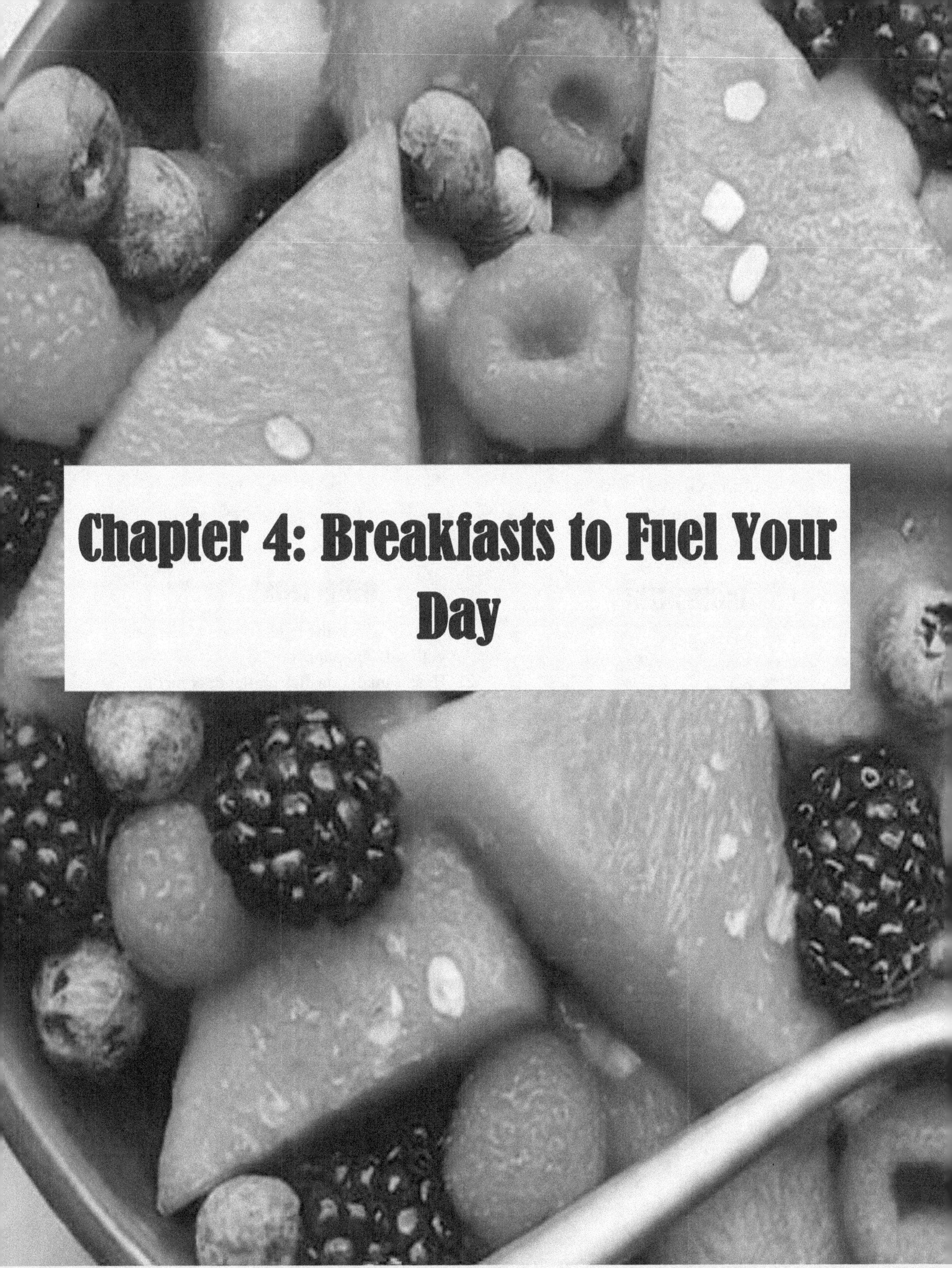

Chapter 4: Breakfasts to Fuel Your Day

Smoked Salmon Scramble

Why We Love It:

- High Protein: Smoked salmon and eggs pack a protein punch, keeping you full and satisfied.
- Omega-3 Power: Smoked salmon delivers heart-healthy omega-3 fatty acids.
- Flavor Boost: The creaminess of Greek yogurt and chives add a fresh, savory twist

Cook Time: *5-7 minutes* ***Prep Time:*** *5 minutes*

Approximate Nutrition Info (per serving):

- Calories: 320
- Protein: 30g
- Carbs: 25g
- Fat: 13g

INGREDIENTS

- 2 large eggs
- 3 ounces smoked salmon, flaked
- 1 tablespoon Greek yogurt
- 1 tablespoon chopped chives
- 1 slice Ezekiel bread
- Salt and black pepper to taste
- Optional: Cooking spray or a touch of olive oil

DIRECTIONS

1. Lightly whisk the eggs in a bowl. Season with salt and pepper.
2. Heat a small nonstick skillet over medium heat. If needed, add a little cooking spray or oil.
3. Pour in the eggs and let them set slightly. Gently scramble them until cooked through.
4. Stir in the smoked salmon and Greek yogurt just before the eggs are fully set.
5. Serve over a slice of toasted Ezekiel bread and garnish with chopped chives.

Tips

- Use fresh dill instead of chives for a flavor variation.
- Add a side of cherry tomatoes or sliced cucumbers for extra

Mighty Protein Bowl

Why We Love It:
- Super Convenient: No cooking required, just layer and go!
- Protein Power-Up: Greek yogurt, cottage cheese, and protein powder combine for a muscle-building boost.
- Customizable: Swap nut butter, protein flavors, and toppings to your liking.

Cook Time: None! **Prep Time:** 2 minutes

Approximate Nutrition Info (per serving):

- Calories: 480
- Protein: 45g
- Carbs: 30g
- Fat: 25g

INGREDIENTS

- ½ cup Greek yogurt
- ½ cup cottage cheese
- 1 scoop protein powder (vanilla or your favorite flavor)
- ¼ cup chopped almonds
- 1 tablespoon natural peanut butter

DIRECTIONS

1. In a bowl, layer the Greek yogurt, cottage cheese, and protein powder.
2. Sprinkle over the chopped almonds.
3. Drizzle with natural peanut butter.

Tips

- Top with berries for extra antioxidants and a touch of sweetness.
- Use a different nut butter, like almond or cashew, if you prefer.

Turkey & Egg Power Wrap

Why We Love It:

- Filling & Portable: A great on-the-go breakfast when you're short on time.
- Lean Protein Focus: Turkey and eggs provide quality protein without added fat.
- Easy to Customize: Add your favorite veggie toppings for extra nutrients.

Cook Time: 5-7 minutes **Prep Time:** 5 minutes

Approximate Nutrition Info (per serving):

- Calories: 280
- Protein: 32g
- Carbs: 20g
- Fat: 10g

INGREDIENTS

- 1 low-carb tortilla
- 3 ounces thinly sliced turkey breast
- 1 large egg
- 1 tablespoon grated low-fat cheese
- Salt and black pepper to taste
- Optional: Cooking spray or a touch of olive oil

DIRECTIONS

1. Lightly whisk the egg in a bowl. Season with salt and pepper.
2. Heat a small nonstick skillet. If needed, add a little cooking spray or oil.
3. Pour in the egg and scramble until cooked through.
4. Warm the tortilla slightly in the microwave or a dry skillet.
5. Lay the turkey on the tortilla, add scrambled egg, and sprinkle with cheese.
6. Roll up tightly. Enjoy immediately.

Tips

- Add chopped spinach or sliced bell peppers to the egg scramble.
- Swap the cheese for a sprinkle of hot sauce for some extra kick!

Lean Beef & Lentil Hash

Why We Love It:

- Hearty & Satisfying: Beef and lentils create a filling combo, great for active mornings.
- Flavorful: Spices like cumin and chili powder liven up this savory dish.
- Make-Ahead Option: Prep the beef and lentil mixture in advance for even faster assembly.

Cook Time: 10-15 minutes Prep Time: 5 minutes (plus lentil cooking time if not pre-cooked)

Approximate Nutritional Info (per serving):

- Calories: 350
- Protein: 35g
- Carbs: 30g
- Fat: 12g

INGREDIENTS

- ½ pound extra-lean ground beef
- ½ cup chopped onion
- 1 cup cooked lentils
- 1 teaspoon cumin
- ½ teaspoon chili powder
- Salt and black pepper to taste
- 1 large egg
- Optional: Cooking spray or a touch of olive oil

DIRECTIONS

1. Heat a large skillet over medium heat. Add a little cooking spray or oil if needed.
2. Add the ground beef and onion. Cook, breaking up the beef, until browned. Drain off any excess fat.
3. Stir in the pre-cooked lentils, cumin, chili powder, salt, and pepper. Cook for a few minutes to warm through.
4. If desired, create a small well in the hash mixture and crack the egg into it. Cover and cook until the egg is set to your liking.

Tips

- Add other chopped veggies like bell peppers or mushrooms for extra nutrients.
- Top with a dollop of salsa or hot sauce for a flavor boost.

Turkey & Egg Power Wrap

Why We Love It:

- Filling & Portable: A great on-the-go breakfast when you're short on time.
- Lean Protein Focus: Turkey and eggs provide quality protein without added fat.
- Easy to Customize: Add your favorite veggie toppings for extra nutrients.

Cook Time: 5-7 minutes **Prep Time:** 5 minutes

Approximate Nutrition Info (per serving):

- Calories: 280
- Protein: 32g
- Carbs: 20g
- Fat: 10g

INGREDIENTS

- 1 low-carb tortilla
- 3 ounces thinly sliced turkey breast
- 1 large egg
- 1 tablespoon grated low-fat cheese
- Salt and black pepper to taste
- Optional: Cooking spray or a touch of olive oil

DIRECTIONS

7. Lightly whisk the egg in a bowl. Season with salt and pepper.
8. Heat a small nonstick skillet. If needed, add a little cooking spray or oil.
9. Pour in the egg and scramble until cooked through.
10. Warm the tortilla slightly in the microwave or a dry skillet.
11. Lay the turkey on the tortilla, add scrambled egg, and sprinkle with cheese.
12. Roll up tightly. Enjoy immediately.

Tips

- Add chopped spinach or sliced bell peppers to the egg scramble.
- Swap the cheese for a sprinkle of hot sauce for some extra kick!

Protein Berry Parfait

Why We Love It:

- Creamy & Sweet: Feels like an indulgence while being packed with healthy ingredients.
- Antioxidant Boost: Berries deliver a powerful dose of antioxidants.
- Quick Assembly: Perfect for when you're pressed for time.

Cook Time: 5-7 minutes **Prep Time:** 5 minutes

Approximate Nutrition Info (per serving):

- Calories: 280
- Protein: 32g
- Carbs: 20g
- Fat: 10g

INGREDIENTS

- 1 cup Greek yogurt
- 1 scoop protein powder (vanilla or berry flavor)
- 1 cup mixed berries (fresh or frozen)

DIRECTIONS

1. In a glass or bowl, layer half the Greek yogurt, followed by half the protein powder and half the berries.
2. Repeat with the remaining yogurt, protein powder, and berries.

Tips

- Experiment with other berries like raspberries or blackberries.
- Add a sprinkle of granola, chopped nuts, or chia seeds for a little crunch.

Tuna Power Cakes

Why We Love It:
- Fishy Twist: A unique way to get your morning protein and omega-3s.
- Easy to Make: Just a few simple ingredients mix up quickly.
- Savory Start: A nice change of pace from sweet breakfasts.

Cook Time: 6-8 minutes **Prep Time:** 5 minutes

Approximate Nutritional Info (per serving):

- Calories: 250
- Protein: 32g
- Carbs: 5g
- Fat:12g

INGREDIENTS

- 1 (5-ounce) can tuna, drained
- 1 large egg
- 1 tablespoon Greek yogurt
- 2 tablespoons chopped green onion
- Salt and black pepper to taste
- Optional: Cooking spray or a touch of olive oil

DIRECTIONS

1. Combine the tuna, egg, Greek yogurt, and chopped green onion in a bowl. Season with salt and pepper.
2. Heat a large nonstick skillet over medium heat. Add a little cooking spray or oil if needed.
3. Form the tuna mixture into patties (about 3-4 patties). Cook for a few minutes per side, or until golden brown and cooked through.

Tips

- Serve with a dollop of salsa or a squeeze of lemon for extra flavor.
- Add a side of sliced avocado for healthy fats.

Veggie-Packed Omelet

Why We Love It:
- Veggie Power: A great way to sneak in extra vegetables for essential nutrients.
- Customizable: Use your favorite veggie combo for variety.
- Balanced Meal: Combine the omelet with a slice of whole-grain bread for healthy carbs.

Cook Time: 5-7 minutes **Prep Time:** 5 minutes

Approximate Nutritional Info (per serving):

- Calories: 200
- Protein: 20g
- Carbs: 5g
- Fat: 12g

INGREDIENTS

- 2 large eggs
- ¼ cup chopped spinach
- ¼ cup chopped mushrooms
- 1 tablespoon grated low-fat cheese
- Salt and black pepper to taste
- Optional: Cooking spray or a touch of olive oil

DIRECTIONS

1. Whisk the eggs in a bowl and season with salt and pepper.
2. Heat a small nonstick omelet pan or skillet over medium heat. Add a little cooking spray or oil if needed.
3. Add the spinach and mushrooms, sauté for a minute or two until softened.
4. Pour in the eggs and swirl the pan to cover the bottom.
5. As the eggs begin to set, sprinkle over the cheese. Fold the omelet in half.
6. Cook for an additional minute or two, until the eggs are fully set.

Tips

- Get creative! Add chopped bell peppers, onions, or a sprinkle of your favorite herbs.
- Top with a spoonful of salsa, hot sauce, or avocado for extra flavor.

Protein Pancake Powerhouse

Why We Love It:

- Treat Yourself: Pancakes that fit your plan! Satisfies those cravings without the sugar crash.
- Protein Boost: The combo of protein powder, cottage cheese, and egg keeps you feeling full for hours.
- Naturally Sweet Option: Ripe bananas add sweetness without extra sugar.

Cook Time: 10-15 minutes **Prep Time:** 5 minutes

Approximate Nutritional Info (per serving):

- Calories: 300
- Protein: 30g
- Carbs: 35g
- Fat: 10g

INGREDIENTS

- 1 scoop protein powder (vanilla or your favorite flavor)
- ½ cup cottage cheese
- 1 large egg
- 1 ripe banana, mashed
- ¼ teaspoon baking powder
- Optional: Cooking spray or a touch of oil
- Optional toppings: Berries, chopped nuts, a drizzle of natural honey

DIRECTIONS

1. Blend all ingredients until smooth.
2. Heat a large nonstick skillet or griddle over medium heat. Add a little cooking spray or oil if needed.
3. Drop batter by ¼ cupfuls onto the hot skillet. Cook for 2-3 minutes per side, or until golden brown and cooked through.

Tips

- Adjust the sweetness: Add a touch of natural honey or maple syrup to the batter if you prefer sweeter pancakes.
- Experiment with mix-ins: Stir in chopped berries, nuts, or a sprinkling of cinnamon.

Egg White & Quinoa Scramble

Why We Love It:

- Light & Nutritious: Egg whites provide lean protein, quinoa adds fiber and complex carbs.
- Boost Your Veggies: Easily toss in plenty of vegetables to amplify the nutrients.
- Savory & Satisfying: Hot sauce adds a little zing to keep things interesting.

Cook Time: 8-10 minutes **Prep Time:** 5 minutes

Approximate Nutritional Info (per serving):

- Calories: 250
- Protein: 25g
- Carbs: 30g
- Fat: 5g

INGREDIENTS

- ½ cup cooked quinoa
- ½ cup chopped bell pepper (any color)
- 1 cup egg whites
- 1 tablespoon hot sauce (or to taste)
- Salt and black pepper to taste
- Optional: Cooking spray or a touch of olive oil

DIRECTIONS

1. Heat a large nonstick skillet over medium heat. Add a little cooking spray or oil if needed.
2. Sauté the bell pepper for a few minutes until softened.
3. Stir in the pre-cooked quinoa and heat through.
4. Pour in the egg whites, scrambling them as they cook.
5. Season with hot sauce, salt, and pepper.

Tips

- Add other veggies of your choice: Spinach, mushrooms, or onions work well.
- Top with a sprinkle of cheese or a dollop of salsa for extra flavor.

Peanut Butter Protein Oats

Why We Love It:
- Classic & Comforting: Warm oats are a satisfying start to any day.
- Protein Punch: Protein powder + peanut butter amp up the fullness factor.
- Flavorful & Filling: Chopped nuts add satisfying crunch.

Cook Time: 5-7 minutes (stovetop) or 2-3 minutes (microwave) **Prep Time:** 2 minutes

Approximate Nutritional Info (per serving):

- Calories: 400
- Protein: 25g
- Carbs: 55g
- Fat: 15g

INGREDIENTS

- ½ cup rolled oats
- 1 cup milk (or unsweetened alternative like almond milk)
- 1 scoop protein powder (vanilla or chocolate work great)
- 1 tablespoon peanut butter
- 1 tablespoon chopped nuts

Tips

- Use your favorite type of nut butter: almond, cashew, or even sunflower seed butter works!
- Add a touch of cinnamon or vanilla extract for extra flavor.

DIRECTIONS

1. **Microwave Method:** Combine oats, milk, and protein powder in a microwave-safe bowl. Microwave on high for 1-2 minutes, or until cooked through. Stir in peanut butter and top with nuts.

2. **Stovetop Method:** Combine oats and milk in a small saucepan. Bring to a simmer over medium heat, stirring occasionally. Cook until oats are tender and thickened. Stir in protein powder and peanut butter. Top with nuts.

Cottage Cheese & Fruit Delight

Why We Love It:

- Simple & Refreshing: The perfect light breakfast option or healthy snack.
- Protein + Fiber: Cottage cheese delivers protein, while the fruit adds fiber and sweetness.
- Fun Toppings: Get creative with nuts, seeds, and spices for variety.

Cook Time: None! **Prep Time:** 2 minutes

Approximate Nutritional Info (per serving):

- Calories: 300
- Protein: 28g
- Carbs: 30g
- Fat: 10g

INGREDIENTS

- 1 cup cottage cheese
- 1 cup mixed berries
- 1 tablespoon chopped nuts
- 1 teaspoon pumpkin seeds
- Sprinkle of cinnamon (optional)

DIRECTIONS

1. Top a bowl of cottage cheese with mixed berries, chopped nuts, and pumpkin seeds. Add a sprinkle of cinnamon if desired.

Tips

- Swap in other fruits: Try sliced peaches, mangoes, or chopped apples.
- Add a tiny drizzle of honey or maple syrup for extra sweetness if needed.

Shellfish Scramble

Why We Love It:

- Sophisticated Twist: A unique and elegant way to elevate your morning eggs.
- Omega-3 Boost: Shellfish like shrimp or scallops provide beneficial fatty acids.
- Flavorful: Garlic, spinach, and a touch of lemon add brightness.

Cook Time: 5-7 minutes **Prep Time:** 5 minutes

Approximate Nutritional Info (per serving):

- Calories: 280
- Protein: 30g
- Carbs: 7g
- Fat: 15g

INGREDIENTS

- 4 ounces peeled and cooked shrimp or scallops
- 1 tablespoon olive oil
- 1 clove garlic, minced
- ½ cup chopped spinach
- 2 large eggs
- Squeeze of fresh lemon juice
- Salt and black pepper to taste

DIRECTIONS

1. Heat the olive oil in a skillet over medium heat. Add garlic and sauté for 30 seconds.
2. Add the shrimp or scallops and spinach. Cook for a minute or two until warmed through.
3. Whisk the eggs with salt and pepper. Pour them into the skillet and scramble.
4. Finish with a squeeze of lemon juice just before serving.

Tips

- Use leftover cooked shellfish to save prep time.
- Add a sprinkle of red pepper flakes for a bit of heat.

Chapter 5: Lunches That Satisfy

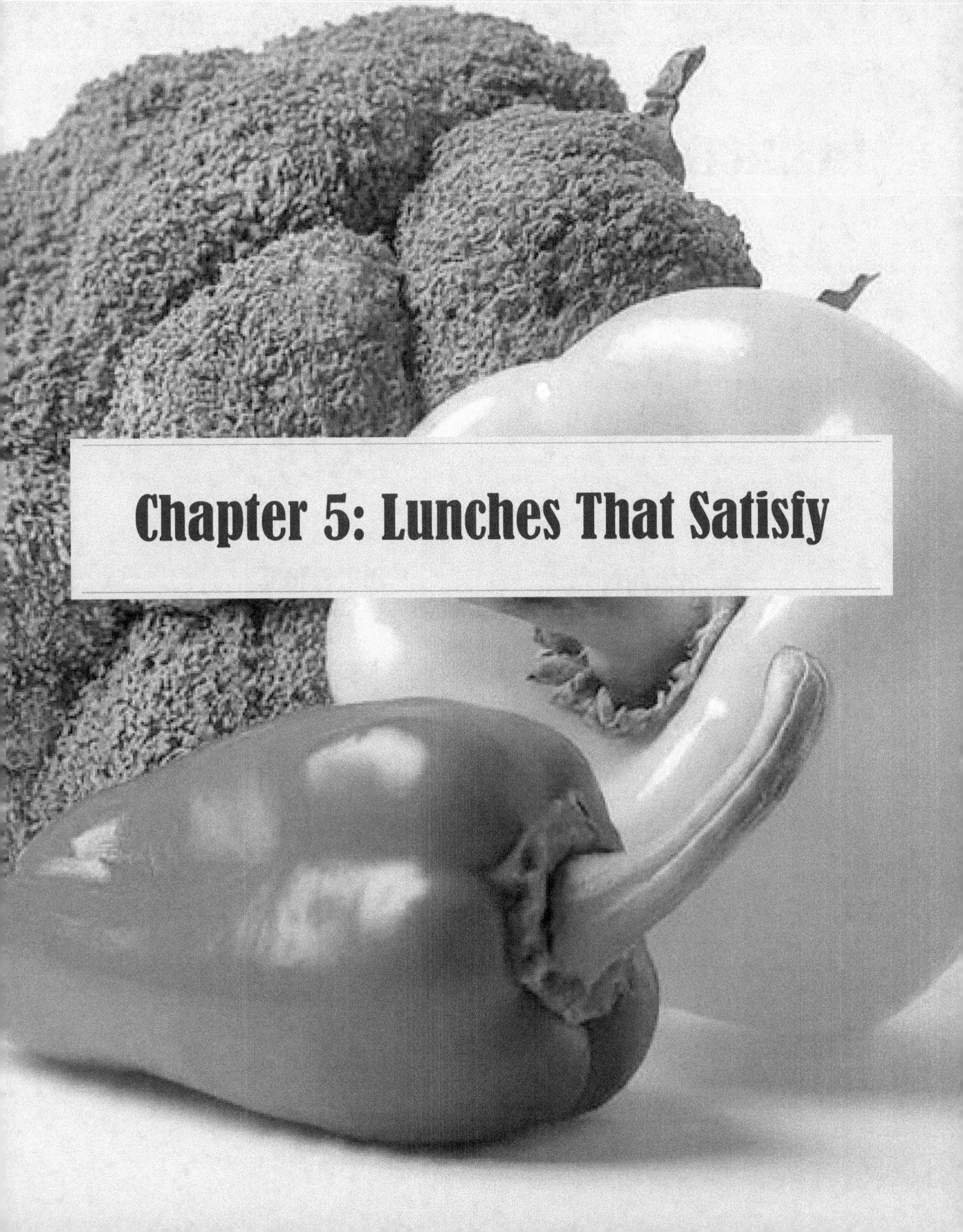

Mediterranean Tuna Power Salad

Why We Love It:
- Classic Flavors: This combo of tuna, olives, feta, and tangy dressing is always a hit.
- Packed with Protein: Tuna delivers a hefty dose to keep those hunger pangs at bay.
- Healthy Fats: Olives, feta (in moderation), and the dressing provide good fats for lasting energy.

Cook Time: None! **Prep Time:** 10 minutes

Approximate Nutritional Info (per serving):

- Calories: 300
- Protein: 25g
- Carbs: 15g
- Fat: 18g

INGREDIENTS

- 1 (5-ounce) can tuna, drained
- ½ cup chopped cucumber
- ½ cup chopped tomato
- ¼ cup sliced black olives
- 2 tablespoons crumbled feta cheese
- 2 tablespoons lemon vinaigrette dressing
- 1-2 cups mixed greens

DIRECTIONS

1. In a bowl, combine the tuna, cucumber, tomato, olives, and feta cheese.
2. Add the lemon vinaigrette and toss to coat.
3. Serve over a bed of mixed greens.

Tips

- Make your own vinaigrette: Whisk olive oil, lemon juice, a bit of Dijon mustard, oregano, salt, and pepper.
- Add other Mediterranean accents like chopped artichoke hearts or capers.

Chicken Quinoa Fiesta

Why We Love It:
- Flavor Explosion: Zesty lime, cilantro, and the sweetness of corn create a vibrant dish.
- Fiber-rich: Quinoa and black beans provide filling fiber for stable blood sugar.
- Make-Ahead Friendly: Prepare the quinoa, chicken, and dressing in advance for quick assembly.

Cook Time: None if chicken and quinoa are pre-cooked **Prep Time:** 15 minutes

Approximate Nutritional Info (per serving):

- Calories: 450
- Protein: 30g
- Carbs: 55g
- Fat: 18g

INGREDIENTS

- 1 cup cooked shredded chicken
- 1 cup cooked quinoa
- ½ cup canned black beans, rinsed and drained
- ½ cup corn (fresh or frozen)
- ½ cup diced bell pepper (any color)
- ¼ cup chopped avocado
- ¼ cup cilantro-lime dressing

Cilantro-Lime Dressing:

- ¼ cup olive oil
- ¼ cup lime juice
- 1 tablespoon chopped cilantro
- Pinch of cumin
- Salt and pepper to taste

DIRECTIONS

1. Make the dressing: Whisk together the dressing ingredients.
2. Combine the chicken, quinoa, black beans, corn, bell pepper, avocado, and cilantro-lime dressing in a bowl. Toss to coat.

Tips

- Use leftover rotisserie chicken for easy prep.
- Add a kick of heat with a dash of hot sauce or chopped jalapeño.

Lentil & Egg Super Salad

Why We Love It:

- Vegetarian Option: Lentils + eggs = plenty of protein without meat.
- Extra Nutritious: Sunflower seeds add a boost of healthy fats and vitamins.
- Simple & Satisfying: A well-balanced salad that's easy to assemble.

Cook Time: None if lentils are pre-cooked **Prep Time:** 10 minutes (plus hard-boiling the eggs)

Approximate Nutritional Info (per serving):

- Calories: 350
- Protein: 25g
- Carbs: 30g
- Fat: 18g

INGREDIENTS

- 1 cup cooked lentils
- 2 hard-boiled eggs, chopped
- 1 cup chopped spinach
- ¼ cup sunflower seeds
- 2 tablespoons balsamic vinaigrette dressing
- Salt and pepper to taste

DIRECTIONS

1. Combine the lentils, hard-boiled eggs, spinach, and sunflower seeds in a bowl.
2. Drizzle with balsamic vinaigrette and toss to coat.
3. Season with salt and pepper.

Tips

- Swap balsamic vinaigrette for your favorite dressing for variety.
- Add other chopped veggies for extra nutrients: cucumbers, tomatoes, etc.

Greek Shrimp & Feta Salad:

Why We Love It:

- Classic Mediterranean Flavors: The combo of tangy feta, briny olives, and a zesty dressing transports you to a seaside taverna.
- Protein-Packed: Shrimp provides lean protein to keep you satisfied.
- Light & Refreshing: Perfect for a warm day or a lighter meal.

INGREDIENTS

Salad Base:

- 4 cups mixed greens (romaine, spinach, arugula, etc.)
- ½ cup chopped cucumber
- ½ cup chopped tomato
- ¼ cup sliced Kalamata olives

Shrimp:

- 1 pound medium shrimp, peeled and deveined
- 1 tablespoon olive oil
- 1 teaspoon dried oregano
- ½ teaspoon garlic powder
- salt and black pepper to taste
- **Feta:** ¼ cup crumbled feta cheese

Greek-Style Dressing:

- ¼ cup olive oil
- 2 tablespoons red wine vinegar
- 1 tablespoon lemon juice
- 1 teaspoon dried oregano
- ½ teaspoon garlic powder
- Salt and pepper to taste

Cook Time: 10 minutes for shrimp **Prep Time:** 15 minutes

Approximate Nutritional Info (per serving): Calories: 350, ● Fat: 22g

- Protein: 30g. Carbs: 15g

DIRECTIONS

1. **Cook the Shrimp:** Toss the shrimp with olive oil, oregano, garlic powder, salt, and pepper. Grill or pan-sear for 2-3 minutes per side, or until cooked through (pink and opaque). Set aside.

2. **Make the Dressing:** Whisk together all dressing ingredients in a small bowl.

3. **Assemble the Salad:** Divide the mixed greens among serving plates. Top with chopped cucumbers, tomatoes, and olives. Add the cooked shrimp and sprinkle with feta cheese.

4. **Dress & Enjoy:** Drizzle with the Greek-style dressing and enjoy immediately!

Tips

- Use leftover grilled shrimp to save on cooking time.
- Add other Greek-inspired ingredients like chopped bell peppers, artichoke hearts, or a sprinkle of capers.
- Serve with a side of whole-wheat pita bread for dipping into the dressing.

Turkey & Hummus Power Wrap

Why We Love It:

- Protein + Fiber: The combo of turkey and hummus delivers both for lasting fullness.
- Flavorful & Fresh: The veggies and mustard add satisfying flavor and crunch.
- Easy to Adapt: Swap the turkey for grilled chicken or use your favorite hummus flavor.

Cook Time: None! **Prep Time:** 5 minutes

Approximate Nutritional Info (per wrap):

- Calories: 350
- Protein: 30g
- Carbs: 40g
- Fat: 15g

INGREDIENTS

- 1 whole-wheat tortilla
- 2-3 tablespoons hummus
- 4 oz sliced turkey breast
- ½ cup spinach
- ¼ cup sliced cucumber
- 1 teaspoon Dijon mustard (optional)

DIRECTIONS

1. Spread the hummus evenly onto the tortilla.
2. Layer with the turkey, spinach, and cucumber. Drizzle with mustard if desired.
3. Roll the tortilla tightly and cut in half if desired.

Tips

- Use flavored hummus like roasted red pepper for an extra flavor boost.
- Add other veggie toppings like shredded carrots or sprouts.

Buffalo Chicken Lettuce Wraps

Why We Love It:

- Spicy & Satisfying: A healthier spin on a favorite appetizer!
- Low Carb Winner: Lettuce wraps keep things light and fresh.
- Quick & Easy: Great for using leftover chicken.

Cook Time: None if chicken is pre-cooked **Prep Time:** 5 minutes

Approximate Nutritional Info (per 2 lettuce wraps):

- Calories: 200
- Protein: 25g
- Carbs: 5g
- Fat: 10g

INGREDIENTS

- 1 cup cooked shredded chicken
- ¼ cup hot sauce
- 1 tablespoon Greek yogurt
- 4-6 large lettuce leaves (Boston or butter lettuce works well)
- Crumbled blue cheese (optional)

DIRECTIONS

1. Combine shredded chicken, hot sauce, and Greek yogurt in a bowl.
2. Place a generous spoonful of chicken mixture into each lettuce leaf.
3. Top with crumbled blue cheese if desired.

Tips

- Adjust the hot sauce level to your desired spice level.
- Add other veggie toppings like diced celery or shredded carrots for extra crunch.

Black Bean Veggie Wrap

Why We Love It:

- Vegetarian Delight: A satisfying and flavorful meatless option.
- Packed with Fiber: Both black beans and veggies deliver filling fiber.
- Healthy Fats: Avocado provides good fats for lasting energy and nutrient absorption.

Cook Time: None! **Prep Time:** 10-15 minutes

Approximate Nutritional Info (per wrap):

- Calories: 380
- Protein: 15g
- Carbs: 55g
- Fat: 15g

INGREDIENTS

- 1 (15-ounce) can black beans, rinsed and drained
- ½ ripe avocado
- 1 teaspoon lime juice
- ¼ teaspoon cumin
- ¼ teaspoon chili powder
- Salt and pepper to taste
- 1 whole-wheat tortilla
- ¼ cup chopped bell pepper (any color)
- ¼ cup chopped onion
- 2 tablespoons salsa

Tips

- Add a squeeze of fresh lime just before serving for extra brightness.
- Get creative with toppings: Try adding shredded lettuce, sliced jalapenos, or a dollop of Greek yogurt.
- Flavor Boost: A sprinkle of hot sauce adds a kick, or try a smoky chipotle seasoning blend mixed into the black beans.

DIRECTIONS

1. **Make the Black Bean Mash:** In a medium bowl, mash black beans with the avocado, lime juice, cumin, chili powder, salt, and pepper. You can leave some beans slightly chunky for texture or create a smoother consistency.
2. **Prep the Veggies:** While mashing the beans, chop the bell peppers and onion into small pieces.
3. **Assemble the Wrap:**
   - Warm the tortilla slightly in a dry skillet or microwave (this makes it more pliable).
   - Spread the black bean mash evenly onto the tortilla.
   - Top with chopped bell pepper, onion, and salsa.
4. **Roll & Enjoy:** Roll the tortilla tightly. You can cut it in half for easier handling if desired. Serve immediately!

Spicy Lentil & Chicken Soup

Why We Love It:

- Hearty & Warming: Perfect for chilly days when you need something substantial.
- Flavor Packed: Spices like cumin and chili powder give it a kick without being overwhelmingly spicy.
- Protein Boost: The combo of lentils and chicken keeps you satisfied.

Cook Time: 20-25 minutes **Prep Time:** 10 minutes

Approximate Nutritional Info (per serving):

- Calories: 280
- Protein: 30g
- Carbs: 30g
- Fat: 8g

INGREDIENTS

- 1 tablespoon olive oil
- ½ cup chopped onion
- 1 clove garlic, minced
- 1 teaspoon cumin
- ½ teaspoon chili powder
- 1 cup cooked lentils
- 1 cup cooked shredded chicken
- 1 (14.5-ounce) can diced tomatoes
- 4 cups chicken or vegetable broth
- Salt and pepper to taste

DIRECTIONS

1. Heat olive oil in a large pot over medium heat. Add onion and cook until softened, about 5 minutes. Stir in garlic and spices and cook for an additional 30 seconds.
2. Add lentils, chicken, diced tomatoes, and broth. Bring to a simmer.
3. Reduce heat and simmer for 15-20 minutes, or until flavors have blended. Season with salt and pepper.

Tips

- Add other chopped veggies like carrots or celery for extra nutrients.
- Top with a dollop of Greek yogurt or a squeeze of lemon for added flavor.

Creamy White Bean & Spinach Soup.

Why We Love It:

- Creamy (Without the Cream!): Blending white beans creates a velvety texture without added dairy fat.
- Super Nutritious: Spinach adds iron, fiber, and vitamins, while white beans provide protein and fiber.
- Easy to Customize: Get creative with flavor additions to make it your own.

INGREDIENTS

- 1 tablespoon olive oil
- ½ cup chopped onion
- 2 cloves garlic, minced
- 1 (15-ounce) can white beans (cannellini or Great Northern), rinsed and drained
- 5 cups baby spinach
- 4 cups vegetable broth
- ¼ cup plain Greek yogurt
- Salt and pepper to taste
- Optional Toppings: Crumbled feta, chopped herbs, a drizzle of olive oil

Tips

- Use a low-sodium vegetable broth to control saltiness.
- Add a pinch of red pepper flakes for a slight kick.
- For a richer flavor, substitute a portion of the vegetable broth with chicken broth.
- Fresh herbs: Top your soup with chopped basil, chives, or parsley for a flavor boost!

Cook Time: 15-20 minutes **Prep Time:** 10 minutes

Approximate Nutritional Info (per serving):

- Calories: 250
- Protein: 15g
- Carbs: 35g
- Fat: 10g

DIRECTIONS

1. **Sauté the Aromatics:** Heat olive oil in a large pot over medium heat. Add onion and cook until softened, about 5 minutes. Add the garlic and cook for an additional 30 seconds, stirring constantly.

2. **Add Beans, Spinach & Broth:** Add the white beans, spinach, and vegetable broth to the pot. Bring to a simmer, then reduce heat and let simmer for 5-10 minutes, or until spinach is wilted.

3. **Blend Until Smooth:** Remove the soup from heat. Using an immersion blender (or carefully transferring to a regular blender in batches), blend the soup until smooth.

4. **Stir in Greek Yogurt:** Once the soup is smooth, stir in the Greek yogurt for extra creaminess and a tangy flavor. Season with salt and pepper to taste.

Cottage Cheese Delight

Why We Love It:
- Super Simple: Minimal prep required, perfect for busy days.
- Balanced Nutrition: Protein from cottage cheese, fiber and sweetness from berries, healthy fats from nuts.

Cook Time: None! **Prep Time:** 2 minutes

Approximate Nutritional Info (per serving):

- Calories: 320
- Protein: 30g
- Carbs: 30g
- Fat: 12g

INGREDIENTS

- 1 cup cottage cheese
- ½ cup mixed berries
- 2 tablespoons chopped nuts
- Drizzle of honey (optional)

DIRECTIONS

1. Top a serving of cottage cheese with mixed berries and chopped nuts.
2. Drizzle with honey if desired.

Tips

- Experiment with different nuts or seeds for variety (walnuts, almonds, pumpkin seeds).
- Swap honey for a sprinkle of cinnamon for a different flavor profile.

Salmon Quinoa Bowl

Why We Love It:

- Omega-3 Powerhouse: Salmon is full of those good-for-you fats that support heart and brain health.
- Balanced & Filling: Quinoa provides complex carbs and fiber for steady energy.
- Versatile: Customize with your favorite veggies and toppings.

Cook Time: 10-15 minutes for salmon, a few minutes to steam broccoli (if not using pre-cooked) **Prep Time:** 5 minutes for dressing + assembly

Approximate Nutritional Info (per bowl):

- Calories: 550
- Protein: 35g
- Carbs: 50g
- Fat: 30g

INGREDIENTS

- 1 cup cooked quinoa
- 4-ounce salmon fillet, cooked
- 1 cup steamed broccoli florets
- ½ avocado, sliced
- Drizzle of lemon-tahini dressing

Lemon-Tahini Dressing:

- ¼ cup tahini
- 2 tablespoons lemon juice
- 1 tablespoon olive oil
- 1 tablespoon water (more as needed for desired consistency)
- Pinch of salt, pepper, and garlic powder

DIRECTIONS

1. Make the dressing: Whisk together tahini, lemon juice, olive oil, water, and spices until smooth.
2. Assemble the bowl: Divide quinoa among serving bowls. Top with cooked salmon, steamed broccoli, and avocado slices.
3. Drizzle with lemon-tahini dressing.

Tips

- Use leftover cooked salmon or rotisserie chicken for easy prep.
- Swap broccoli for any other steamed or roasted veggie you like.

Tex-Mex Beef Power Bowl

Why We Love It:

- Taco-Inspired Flavor: All those Tex-Mex favorites in a healthier format.
- Make It Spicy: Amp up the heat with jalapeños or your favorite hot sauce.
- Make-Ahead Option: Ground beef cooks quickly, but can also be prepped in advance.

Cook Time: 10-15 minutes **Prep Time:** 5 minutes + assembly

Approximate Nutritional Info (per bowl):

- Calories: 500
- Protein: 35g
- Carbs: 60g
- Fat: 15g

INGREDIENTS

- 1 cup cooked brown rice or quinoa
- ½ pound lean ground beef
- 1 teaspoon taco seasoning
- ½ cup canned black beans, rinsed and drained
- ½ cup salsa
- ¼ cup shredded reduced-fat cheddar cheese (optional)
- Dollop of plain Greek yogurt (instead of sour cream)

DIRECTIONS

1. Brown the ground beef in a skillet over medium heat. Drain off any excess fat. Stir in taco seasoning.
2. Assemble the bowl: Divide rice or quinoa among serving bowls. Top with seasoned beef, black beans, and salsa.
3. Finish with a dollop of Greek yogurt and a sprinkle of cheese (if desired).

Tips

- Add chopped lettuce, diced tomatoes, or other toppings for extra freshness.
- Substitute ground turkey or a vegetarian protein alternative if desired.

Asian Tofu Stir-Fry Bowl

Why We Love It:
- Meatless Option: Great for vegetarians or anyone looking to mix up protein sources.
- Flavorful Sauce: Soy-ginger combo gives a classic Asian-inspired taste.
- Veggie-Packed: Great way to boost your daily veggie intake.

Cook Time: 15-20 minutes **Prep Time:** 10 minutes

Approximate Nutritional Info (per bowl):

- Calories: 450
- Protein: 25g
- Carbs: 65g
- Fat: 15g

INGREDIENTS

- 1 cup cooked brown rice
- 14-ounce package firm tofu, pressed and cubed
- 1 tablespoon cornstarch
- 1 tablespoon soy sauce
- 1 teaspoon sesame oil
- 1 teaspoon grated ginger
- 1 cup mixed stir-fry vegetables (broccoli, carrots, snap peas, etc.)

DIRECTIONS

1. Toss tofu cubes with cornstarch.
2. Heat sesame oil in a skillet over medium-high heat. Add tofu and cook until golden brown on all sides. Remove from skillet.
3. Add mixed vegetables and a splash of water to the skillet. Cook until crisp-tender.
4. Return tofu to the skillet. Whisk together soy sauce and ginger, add to the skillet and cook until sauce thickens slightly.
5. Assemble the bowl: Divide cooked rice among bowls. Top with stir-fried tofu and vegetables.

Tips

- Use your favorite pre-made stir-fry sauce for ease, but watch for added sugars.
- Add a sprinkle of sesame seeds or chopped green onions for garnish.

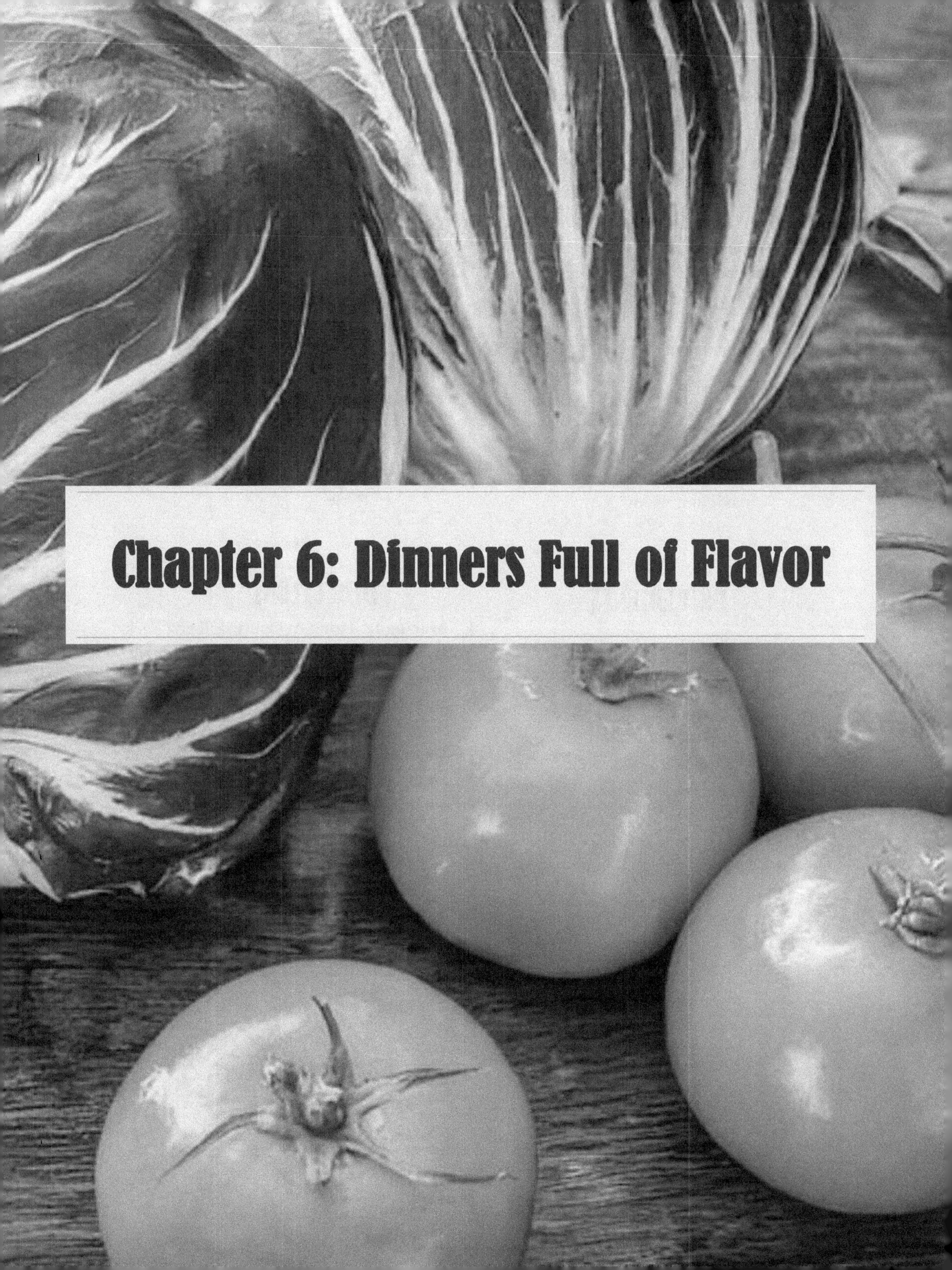
Chapter 6: Dinners Full of Flavor

Greek Yogurt Marinated Chicken

Why We Love It:

- Super Tender & Juicy: The enzymes in yogurt tenderize the chicken, while the tanginess adds flavor.
- Easy to Customize: Experiment with your favorite herbs and spices.
- Make-Ahead: Let the chicken marinate overnight for maximum flavor.

Cook Time: Varies by method. 5-7 minutes per side on grill, 20-25 minutes baking. **Prep Time:** 10 minutes + marinating time

Approximate Nutritional Info (per serving):

- Calories: 250
- Protein: 35g
- Carbs: 5g
- Fat: 12g

INGREDIENTS

- 2 boneless, skinless chicken breasts (or 4 chicken thighs)
- 1 cup plain Greek yogurt
- 2 tablespoons lemon juice
- 1 tablespoon olive oil
- 1 teaspoon dried oregano (or other herbs like thyme, rosemary)
- 1 clove garlic, minced
- Salt and pepper to taste

Tips

- Use a meat thermometer to ensure the chicken is fully cooked.
- Leftovers are great! Slice for salads, wraps, or quesadillas.

DIRECTIONS

1. **Marinade Time:** Whisk together Greek yogurt, lemon juice, olive oil, oregano, garlic, salt, and pepper in a bowl or ziplock bag. Add chicken, coating thoroughly. Marinate in the refrigerator for at least 30 minutes, or ideally several hours or overnight.
2. **Cook Your Way:**
   - Grill: Preheat grill to medium-high heat. Grill chicken for 5-7 minutes per side, or until cooked through (internal temperature reaches 165°F).
   - Bake: Preheat oven to 400°F. Place chicken on a baking sheet, bake for 20-25 minutes or until cooked through.

Spicy Peanut Chicken Stir-Fry

Why We Love It:

- Flavor Explosion: Sweet, spicy, and savory for a satisfying meal.
- Veggie Packed: Easy way to sneak in extra vegetables.
- Quick & Easy: Ready in under 30 minutes, perfect for busy evenings.

INGREDIENTS

- 1 pound boneless, skinless chicken breast, cut into cubes
- 1 tablespoon cornstarch
- 2 tablespoons vegetable oil
- 1 cup broccoli florets
- 1 red bell pepper, sliced
- ½ cup carrots, sliced
- Salt and pepper to taste

Peanut Sauce:

- ¼ cup natural peanut butter
- 2 tablespoons soy sauce (or tamari for gluten-free)
- 1 tablespoon rice vinegar
- 1 tablespoon honey
- 1 clove garlic, minced
- 1 teaspoon grated ginger
- Sriracha (or other hot sauce) to taste

Cook Time: 15-20 minutes **Prep Time:** 15 minutes

Approximate Nutritional Info (per serving):

- Calories: 450
- Protein: 35g
- Carbs: 30g
- Fat: 25g

DIRECTIONS

1. **Prep & Sauce:** Toss chicken with cornstarch. Whisk peanut sauce ingredients together.
2. **Stir-Fry!:** Heat 1 tablespoon oil in a large skillet or wok over high heat. Add chicken in a single layer, cook until browned (don't overcrowd the pan!). Remove to a plate.
3. **Veggie Time:** Add remaining oil to skillet. Stir-fry broccoli, bell pepper, and carrots until crisp-tender.
4. **Finish It:** Add cooked chicken back. Pour in peanut sauce. Cook, stirring, until sauce thickens and coats everything.

Tips

- Swap chicken for shrimp or tofu for variations.
- Add other stir-fry veggies: snap peas, baby corn, etc.
- Garnish with chopped peanuts and cilantro for extra flavor.

Chicken & Lentil Fiesta

Why We Love It:

- One-Pot Wonder: Minimal cleanup, maximum flavor!
- Warming & Cozy: Perfect for chilly nights.
- Easy to Adjust: Customize with your favorite toppings.

Cook Time: 30-35 minutes **Prep Time:** 10 minutes

Approximate Nutritional Info (per serving):

- Calories: 350
- Protein: 35g
- Carbs: 40g
- Fat: 10g

INGREDIENTS

- 1 tablespoon olive oil
- ½ cup chopped onion
- 1 cup dry lentils, rinsed
- 4 cups chicken broth
- 1 (14.5-ounce) can diced tomatoes, undrained
- 1 teaspoon cumin
- ½ teaspoon chili powder
- Salt and pepper to taste
- 1 cup cooked shredded chicken
- Topping ideas: Greek yogurt, diced avocado, cilantro, lime wedges

DIRECTIONS

1. Sauté onion in olive oil in a large pot over medium heat until softened.
2. Add lentils, broth, diced tomatoes, cumin, chili powder, salt, and pepper. Bring to a boil, reduce heat, and simmer for 25-30 minutes, or until lentils are tender.
3. Stir in cooked shredded chicken and heat through.
4. Serve hot, topped with your favorite toppings.

Tips

- Use leftover rotisserie chicken for easy prep.
- Add a kick of heat with chopped jalapeño or a pinch of cayenne.

One-Pan Chicken & Quinoa Bake

Why We Love It:
- Complete Meal: Protein, carbs, and veggies all in one dish.
- Easy Cleanup: Minimal dishes equal a happy cook!
- Flavorful & Nourishing: Herbs and broth infuse the quinoa with deliciousness.

Cook Time: 40-50 minutes **Prep Time:** 15 minutes

Approximate Nutritional Info (per serving):

- Calories: 380
- Protein: 35g
- Carbs: 35g
- Fat: 12g

INGREDIENTS

- 1 pound boneless, skinless chicken breasts, cut into cubes
- 1 cup uncooked quinoa, rinsed
- 1 cup chopped zucchini
- 1 cup chopped bell peppers (any color)
- 1 tablespoon olive oil
- 2 cups low-sodium chicken broth
- 1 teaspoon dried Italian seasoning
- ½ teaspoon garlic powder
- Salt and pepper to taste

DIRECTIONS

1. Preheat oven to 375°F. Lightly grease a 9x13 inch baking dish.
2. In a bowl, toss together the chicken, quinoa, zucchini, bell peppers, olive oil, broth, Italian seasoning, garlic powder, salt, and pepper.
3. Pour the mixture into the prepared baking dish. Cover tightly with foil.
4. Bake for 30-35 minutes, then uncover and bake for an additional 10-15 minutes, or until chicken is cooked through and quinoa is tender.

Tips

- Add other chopped veggies: broccoli, carrots, mushrooms work well.
- Swap quinoa for brown rice or another whole grain if you prefer.
- For extra cheesy goodness, sprinkle with some Parmesan cheese during the last few minutes of baking.

Lemon Garlic Salmon & Asparagus

Why We Love It:
- Simple & Elegant: Minimal ingredients with maximum flavor.
- Heart-Healthy: Salmon provides omega-3s, asparagus adds fiber and vitamins.
- Easy One-Pan Meal: Ready in under 30 minutes.

Cook Time: 12-15 minutes **Prep Time:** 10 minutes

Approximate Nutritional Info (per serving):

- Calories: 350
- Protein: 35g
- Carbs: 10g
- Fat: 20g

INGREDIENTS

- 4 (6-ounce) salmon fillets
- 1 pound asparagus, trimmed
- 2 tablespoons olive oil
- 2 cloves garlic, minced
- 2 tablespoons lemon juice
- Salt and pepper to taste

Tips

- Sprinkle with fresh herbs like dill or parsley for extra flavor.
- Serve with a side of brown rice or quinoa for a more complete meal.

DIRECTIONS

1. Preheat oven to 425°F. Line a baking sheet with parchment paper.
2. Toss asparagus with 1 tablespoon olive oil, salt, and pepper. Place on prepared baking sheet.
3. In a small bowl, whisk together remaining olive oil, garlic, and lemon juice. Brush salmon fillets with the mixture.
4. Bake for 12-15 minutes, or until salmon is cooked through (flakes easily with a fork) and asparagus is tender.

Tuna Steak Power Bowl

Why We Love It:
- Protein Powerhouse: Tuna packs a hefty protein punch.
- Customizable: Swap toppings based on what you have on hand.
- Omega-3 Boost: Tuna delivers those heart-healthy fats.

Cook Time: 5-10 minutes for tuna, plus quinoa cook time **Prep Time:** 10 minutes + dressing

Approximate Nutritional Info (per bowl):

- Calories: 550
- Protein: 40g
- Carbs: 55g
- Fat: 25g

INGREDIENTS

- 2 (6-ounce) tuna steaks
- 1 tablespoon olive oil
- Salt and pepper to taste
- 2 cups cooked quinoa
- 2 cups baby spinach
- 1 cup roasted chickpeas (canned, drained and rinsed, or roast your own)

Tahini-Lemon Dressing:
- ¼ cup tahini
- 3 tablespoons lemon juice
- 2 tablespoons water
- 1 clove garlic, minced
- Pinch of salt and pepper

DIRECTIONS

1. **Make the Dressing:** Whisk together tahini, lemon juice, water, garlic, salt, and pepper. Adjust consistency with additional water as desired.
2. **Cook the Tuna:** Season tuna steaks with salt and pepper. Heat olive oil in a skillet over medium-high heat. Sear tuna steaks for 2-3 minutes per side, or to desired doneness.
3. **Assemble the Bowls:** Divide quinoa, spinach, and roasted chickpeas among bowls. Top with sliced tuna and drizzle

Tips

- Use leftover salmon or other grilled fish as a substitute for tuna.
- Add other toppings: sliced avocado, cucumbers, chopped tomatoes, etc.
- For extra spice, drizzle with Sriracha or your favorite hot sauce.

Shrimp Scampi with Zucchini Noodles

Why We Love It:
- Light & Refreshing: A lower-carb alternative to traditional pasta scampi.
- Quick & Easy: Ready in under 20 minutes, perfect for a weeknight meal.
- Classic Flavors: Garlic, white wine, and lemon bring bright, zesty flavors.

Cook Time: 10-15 minutes **Prep Time:** 10 minutes

Approximate Nutritional Info (per serving):

- Calories: 300
- Protein: 30g
- Carbs: 15g
- Fat: 18g

INGREDIENTS

- 1 pound large shrimp, peeled and deveined
- 2 tablespoons olive oil
- 3 cloves garlic, minced
- ½ cup dry white wine
- ¼ cup lemon juice
- Salt and pepper to taste
- 2-3 medium zucchini, spiralized
- ¼ cup chopped fresh parsley (optional)

Tips

- Pat shrimp dry before cooking for better browning.
- Don't overcook shrimp, they'll become rubbery.
- For extra richness, swirl in a pat of butter at the end of cooking.

DIRECTIONS

1. **Spiralize Zucchini:** Use a spiralizer or julienne peeler to create zucchini noodles.
2. **Sauté Shrimp:** Heat olive oil in a large skillet over medium-high heat. Add shrimp and season with salt and pepper. Cook for 2-3 minutes per side, or until pink and opaque. Remove from skillet.
3. **Garlic & Sauce:** Add garlic to the skillet and cook for 30 seconds, stirring constantly. Deglaze the pan with white wine and lemon juice, scraping up any browned bits. Simmer for 1-2 minutes.
4. **Finish it Up:** Add zucchini noodles to the skillet and cook for 1-2 minutes, just until heated through. Stir in cooked shrimp and parsley (if using).

Tofu & Veggie Power Bowl

Why We Love It:
- Protein-Rich: Tofu is an excellent source of plant-based protein.
- Flavorful & Versatile: Adjust the sauce and veggies to your liking.
- Filling & Nourishing: Brown rice and veggies provide fiber and complex carbs.

Cook Time: 15-20 minutes **Prep Time:** 15 minutes

Approximate Nutritional Info (per serving):

- Calories: 500
- Protein: 25g
- Carbs: 70g
- Fat: 18g

INGREDIENTS

- 1 (14-ounce) block firm tofu, pressed and cubed
- 1 tablespoon cornstarch
- 2 tablespoons vegetable oil
- 1 cup broccoli florets
- 1 bell pepper, sliced (any color)
- ½ cup snap peas

Teriyaki-Style Sauce:

- ¼ cup soy sauce (or tamari for gluten-free)
- 2 tablespoons rice vinegar
- 1 tablespoon honey (or maple syrup)
- 1 clove garlic, minced
- 1 teaspoon grated ginger
- Sriracha (or other hot sauce) to taste

DIRECTIONS

1. **Prep the Tofu:** Toss tofu cubes with cornstarch to coat.
2. **Make the Sauce:** Whisk together the teriyaki sauce ingredients.
3. **Cook Time:** Heat 1 tablespoon of oil in a large skillet or wok over high heat. Add tofu, cook until golden brown on all sides. Remove from pan.
4. **Veggie Time:** Add the remaining oil to the skillet. Cook broccoli, bell peppers, and snap peas until crisp-tender.
5. **Finish it Up:** Return tofu to the pan. Pour in the teriyaki sauce and cook, stirring, until sauce thickens and coats everything. Serve over brown rice.

Tips

- Experiment with different sauces: Sweet chili, peanut sauce, or your own creation!
- Add other stir-fry veggies: baby corn, onions, mushrooms, etc.
- Garnish with sesame seeds and green onions for extra flavor and flair.
- Add a side of sliced avocado for healthy fats.

Spicy Black Bean Burgers

Why We Love It:
- Vegetarian Delight: Hearty and satisfying, even meat-eaters will love these!
- Flavor Packed: Spices and oats create amazing texture and taste.
- Make-Ahead Option: Burgers can be prepped in advance and frozen.

Cook Time: 10-15 minutes **Prep Time:** 15 minutes

Approximate Nutritional Info (per burger):

- Calories: 250
- Protein: 15g
- Carbs: 35g
- Fat: 10g

INGREDIENTS

- 1 (15-ounce) can black beans, rinsed and drained
- ½ cup rolled oats
- 1 egg
- ¼ cup chopped onion
- 1 teaspoon chili powder
- 1 teaspoon cumin
- ½ teaspoon garlic powder
- Salt and pepper to taste
- Whole-wheat buns and your favorite toppings

DIRECTIONS

1. **Mash & Mix:** In a bowl, mash black beans (leaving some texture). Add oats, egg, onion, spices, salt and pepper. Mix well.
2. **Form Patties:** Divide the mixture into 4 patties.
3. **Cook 'em Up:** Heat a skillet or grill pan over medium heat. Cook burgers for 4-5 minutes per side, or until heated through.
4. **Build Your Burger:** Serve on whole-wheat buns with toppings like lettuce, tomato, avocado, sliced onion, and your

Tips

- For a smoky flavor, add a pinch of smoked paprika to the burger mixture.
- Top with a dollop of Greek yogurt for a creamy touch.

Lentil & Spinach Curry

Why We Love It:

- Warming & Flavorful: A cozy and fragrant dish packed with spices.
- Budget-Friendly: Lentils are an affordable protein source.
- Easy to Adapt: Adjust the spice level and add your favorite veggies.

Cook Time: 30-35 minutes **Prep Time:** 10 minutes

Approximate Nutritional Info (per serving):

- Calories: 320
- Protein: 20g
- Carbs: 45g
- Fat: 12g

INGREDIENTS

- 1 tablespoon olive oil
- 1 cup chopped onion
- 2 cloves garlic, minced
- 1 tablespoon grated ginger
- 1 teaspoon cumin
- 1 teaspoon coriander
- ½ teaspoon turmeric
- ¼ teaspoon cayenne pepper (or more/less to adjust spice level)
- 1 cup dry lentils, rinsed
- 1 (14.5-ounce) can diced tomatoes, undrained
- 4 cups vegetable broth
- 5 cups baby spinach
- ½ cup unsweetened coconut milk
- Salt and pepper to taste
- Cooked basmati rice or naan bread for serving (optional)

DIRECTIONS

1. **Sauté Aromatics:** Heat olive oil in a large pot over medium heat. Add onion, garlic, and ginger, cook until softened.
2. **Add Spices & Lentils:** Stir in the spices and toast for 30 seconds for fragrant. Then, add lentils, diced tomatoes, and vegetable broth. Bring to a boil, then reduce heat and simmer for 25-30 minutes, or until lentils are tender.
3. **Finish the Curry:** Stir in spinach and coconut milk. Cook for a few minutes until spinach wilts. Season with salt and pepper.
4. **Serve & Enjoy:** Serve hot with cooked basmati rice or naan bread, if desired.

Tips

- Use other lentils: Brown or green lentils work too, may need slightly longer cooking time.
- Add more veggies: Diced carrots, bell peppers, or potatoes would be delicious.
- Garnish with fresh cilantro for a burst of freshness.

Quinoa Stuffed Peppers

Why We Love It:
- Fun & Festive: A colorful, satisfying stuffed pepper presentation.
- Make-Ahead Friendly: Can be assembled in advance and baked later.
- Nutritious: Packed with fiber, protein, and antioxidants.

Cook Time: 20-25 minutes (baking) Prep Time: 20 minutes

Approximate Nutritional Info (per stuffed pepper half):
- **Calories: 300**
- **Protein: 20g**
- **Carbs: 40g**
- **Fat: 12g**

INGREDIENTS

- 4 bell peppers, any color
- 1 tablespoon olive oil
- ½ cup chopped onion
- 1 cup cooked quinoa
- 1 (15-ounce) can black beans, rinsed and drained
- ½ cup corn (fresh or frozen)
- 1 teaspoon chili powder
- ½ teaspoon cumin
- Salt and pepper to taste
- 1 cup shredded cheddar cheese (or your favorite melty cheese)

DIRECTIONS

1. **Prep the Peppers:** Cut bell peppers in half lengthwise, remove seeds and membranes.
2. **Make the Filling:** Heat olive oil in a skillet. Sauté onion until softened. Add cooked quinoa, black beans, corn, spices, salt, and pepper. Cook until heated through.
3. **Stuff & Bake:** Preheat oven to 375°F. Stuff pepper halves with filling. Top with shredded cheese. Bake for 20-25 minutes, or until peppers are tender and cheese is melted and bubbly.

Tips

- Experiment with different fillings: Try adding chopped mushrooms, zucchini, or crumbled tempeh.
- For a spicier kick, add a diced jalapeño to the filling.
- Top with a dollop of Greek yogurt or salsa for extra flavor.

Steak & Egg Powerhouse

Why We Love It:

- Protein Punch: A classic combination for muscle building and sustained energy.
- Simple & Fast: Ready in minutes, perfect for when you're short on time.
- Versatile: Customize with your favorite steak cut and desired doneness.

Cook Time: 10-15 minutes depending on steak thickness and desired doneness
Prep Time: 5 minutes

Approximate Nutritional Info (per serving):

- Calories: 400 (can vary based on steak size)
- Protein: 45g
- Carbs: 5g
- Fat: 25g

INGREDIENTS

- 1 (6-8 ounce) lean steak (sirloin, flank, top round work well)
- 1 tablespoon olive oil
- Salt and black pepper to taste
- 1-2 large eggs
- Steamed broccoli (or your favorite side vegetable)

Tips

- Use a meat thermometer for accurate doneness.
- For extra flavor, marinate steak in your favorite herbs and spices.

DIRECTIONS

1. **Prep & Season:** Pat the steak dry and season generously with salt and pepper.
2. **Cook Steak:** Heat olive oil in a skillet over medium-high heat. Add steak and cook to desired doneness (3-5 minutes per side for medium-rare). Let rest for a few minutes before slicing.
3. **Cook Eggs:** Fry your eggs in the same skillet to your liking (sunny-side-up, over-easy, etc.).
4. **Serve it Up:** Plate the sliced steak, add fried eggs, and a side of steamed broccoli.

Turkey Meatballs & Zucchini Noodles

Why We Love It:

- Healthier Spin on Comfort Food: Zucchini noodles replace pasta for a lighter take.
- Flavorful: Ground turkey absorbs the delicious marinara sauce.
- Make-Ahead Option: Meatballs can be made and frozen in advance.

Cook Time: 20-25 minutes **Prep Time:** 20 minutes

Approximate Nutritional Info (per serving):

- Calories: 450
- Protein: 35g
- Carbs: 30g
- Fat: 25g

INGREDIENTS

- 1 pound lean ground turkey
- ½ cup breadcrumbs (use whole-wheat if preferred)
- 1 egg
- ¼ cup grated Parmesan cheese
- 1 teaspoon dried Italian seasoning
- Salt and pepper to taste
- 2-3 medium zucchini, spiralized
- Your favorite marinara sauce

Tips

- For extra tenderness, soak breadcrumbs in a little milk before adding to meat mixture.
- Use a homemade marinara sauce to control sugar content.

DIRECTIONS

1. **Make Meatballs:** Combine ground turkey, breadcrumbs, egg, Parmesan, Italian seasoning, salt, and pepper in a bowl. Form into meatballs.
2. **Bake 'em Up:** Preheat oven to 400°F. Bake meatballs for 15-20 minutes, or until cooked through.
3. **Cook Zucchini:** In the last few minutes of meatball cooking, briefly sauté zucchini noodles in a skillet with a touch of olive oil or just warm them through in the marinara sauce.
4. **Plate & Enjoy:** Serve meatballs over zucchini noodles with a generous helping of marinara sauce.

Cottage Cheese Lasagna Roll-Ups

Why We Love It:

- Cheesy Goodness: A satisfying alternative to traditional lasagna.
- Lower Carb: Uses lasagna noodles for a lighter, portion-controlled version.
- Protein Packed: Cottage cheese and spinach deliver a protein boost.

Cook Time: 30-35 minutes **Prep Time:** 20 minutes

Approximate Nutritional Info (per 2 roll-ups):

- Calories: 400
- Protein: 30g
- Carbs: 40g
- Fat: 15g

INGREDIENTS

- 12 lasagna noodles, cooked according to package directions
- 1 (15-ounce) container ricotta cheese
- 1 cup cottage cheese
- 1 large egg
- 1 cup chopped spinach, thawed and squeezed dry (frozen works)
- Salt and pepper to taste
- 1 teaspoon dried Italian seasoning
- 2 cups marinara sauce
- ½ cup shredded mozzarella cheese

DIRECTIONS

1. **Make the Filling:** Combine ricotta, cottage cheese, egg, spinach, Italian seasoning, salt, and pepper.
2. **Assemble Roll-Ups:** Spread a thin layer of marinara on the bottom of a 9x13 inch baking dish. Lay out cooked lasagna noodles. Spread a few tablespoons of the cheese filling on each noodle. Roll up carefully. Place seam-side down in the baking dish.
3. **Top & Bake:** Pour remaining marinara over roll-ups. Sprinkle with mozzarella. Cover with foil. Bake at 375°F for 20-25 minutes. Uncover and bake for an additional 5-10 minutes or until bubbly.

Tips

- Use whole-wheat lasagna noodles for extra fiber.
- Add sautéed ground turkey or beef to the filling for a heartier dish.
- Garnish with fresh basil for a burst of flavor.

Eggs in Purgatory

Why We Love It:

- Bold Flavors: Spicy tomato sauce packs a flavor punch.
- One-Pan Wonder: Minimal dishes for easy cleanup.
- Budget-Friendly: Uses simple, pantry-staple ingredients.

Cook Time: 20-25 minutes
Prep Time: 10 minutes

Approximate Nutritional Info (per serving):

- Calories: 350
- Protein: 25g
- Carbs: 25g
- Fat: 20g

INGREDIENTS

- 1 tablespoon olive oil
- ½ cup chopped onion
- 2 cloves garlic, minced
- 1 (28-ounce) can crushed tomatoes
- 1 teaspoon dried oregano
- ½ teaspoon red pepper flakes (adjust for spice level)
- Salt and pepper to taste
- 4-6 large eggs
- Toppings: Grated Parmesan, fresh basil (optional)

Tips

- Spice it up: Add a pinch of cayenne or chopped jalapeño for more heat.
- Get creative with toppings: Try feta cheese, chopped olives, or a drizzle of pesto.

DIRECTIONS

1. **Make the Sauce:** Heat olive oil in a large skillet over medium heat. Sauté onion until softened. Add garlic and cook for 30 seconds. Stir in crushed tomatoes, oregano, red pepper flakes, salt, and pepper. Simmer for 15 minutes, or until sauce thickens slightly.
2. **Crack the Eggs:** Create small wells in the sauce and carefully crack an egg into each well.
3. **Cook & Finish:** Reduce heat to low, cover, and cook until egg whites are set but yolks are still runny (adjust cooking time for desired doneness). Top with Parmesan and fresh basil if desired. Serve hot with crusty bread for dipping (whole wheat, if preferred).

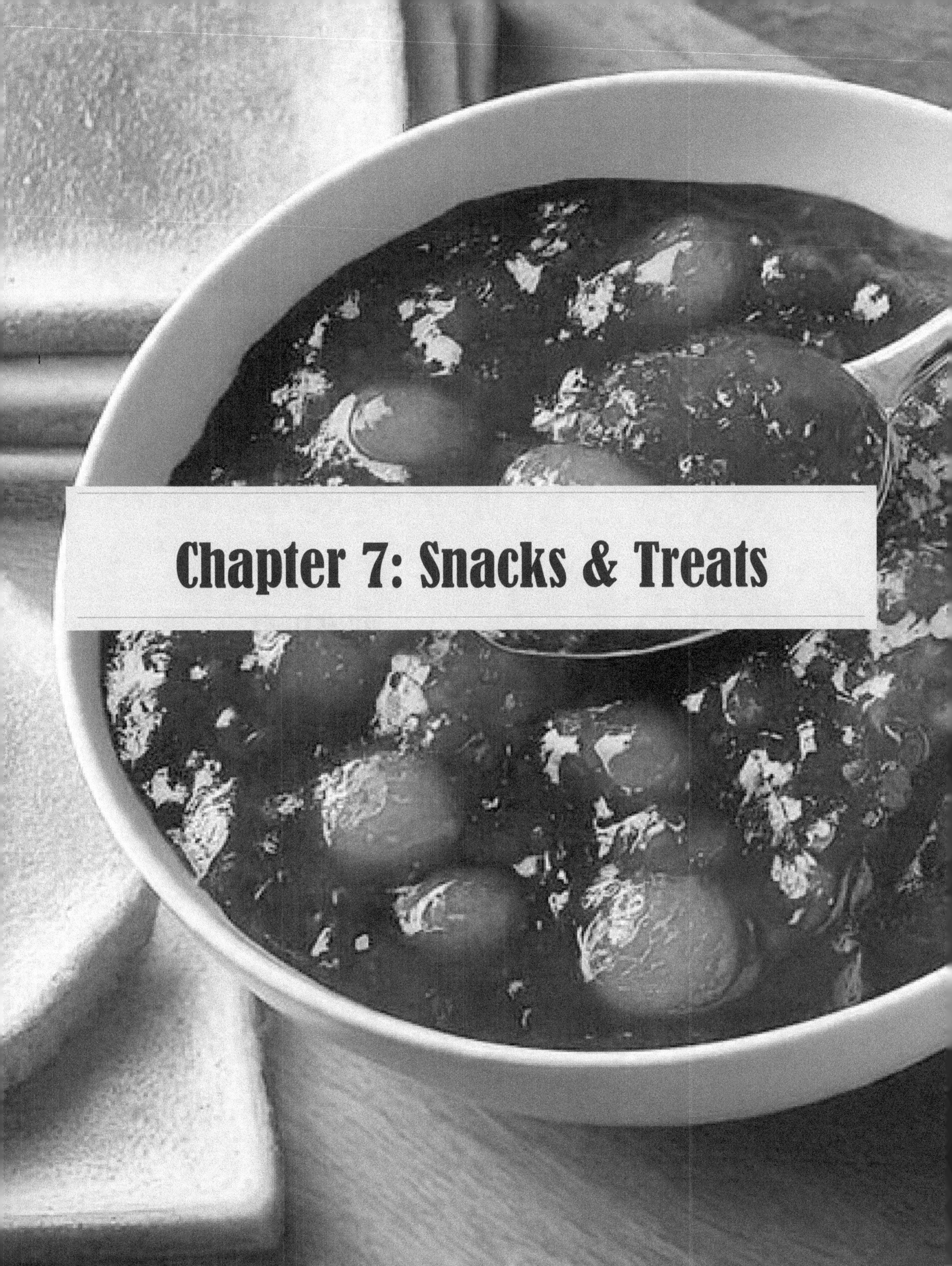
Chapter 7: Snacks & Treats

Greek Yogurt Dip & Veggie Sticks

Why We Love It:
- Super Fresh: Crunchy veggies + creamy, tangy dip = perfect combo.
- Customizable: Get creative with your favorite herbs and spices.
- High in Protein: Greek yogurt delivers that protein punch.

Prep Time: 5 minutes **Cook Time:** None!

Approximate Nutritional Info (per serving of dip + veggies):

- Calories: 100
- Protein: 10g
- Carbs: 10g
- Fat: 3g

INGREDIENTS

- 1 cup plain Greek yogurt
- 1 tablespoon chopped fresh herbs (dill, chives, parsley, etc., or a combination)
- ½ teaspoon lemon juice
- Salt and pepper to taste
- Sliced vegetables: cucumbers, carrots, bell peppers, celery, etc.

DIRECTIONS

1. Whisk together the Greek yogurt, herbs, lemon juice, salt, and pepper.
2. Cut the vegetables into sticks or slices for dipping.
3. Serve the dip alongside your favorite veggies.

Tips

- Add a pinch of garlic powder or onion powder for extra flavor.
- Experiment with different vegetables like radishes, snap peas, or cherry tomatoes.

Hard-Boiled Egg Power Bites

Why We Love It:
- Classic & Simple: Hard-boiled eggs are a perfect no-fuss snack.
- Protein Packed: A single egg provides around 6 grams of protein.
- Portable: Perfect for on-the-go fuel.

Prep Time: 5 minutes (plus hard-boiling time) **Cook Time:** Varies depending on how you boil your eggs.

Approximate Nutritional Info (per large egg):

- Calories: 70
- Protein: 6g
- Carbs: 0.5g
- Fat: 5g

INGREDIENTS

- Hard-boiled eggs
- Your favorite seasonings: salt, pepper, smoked paprika, everything bagel seasoning, etc.

DIRECTIONS

1. Hard boil your eggs to your desired yolk consistency. Let cool completely.
2. Peel and slice or cut into halves.
3. Sprinkle with your favorite seasoning.

Tips

- Bulk prep: Hard boil a batch of eggs at the start of the week for grab-and-go snacks.
- Change it up: Try a sprinkle of curry powder or a dash of hot sauce.

Tuna Cucumber Boats

Why We Love It:

- Low-Carb & Refreshing: Cucumber provides a satisfying crunch.
- Easy to Make: No cooking required, minimal prep!
- Protein Boost: Tuna delivers a good dose of protein and omega-3s.

Prep Time: 10 minutes **Cook Time:** None!

Approximate Nutritional Info (per 2 stuffed cucumber halves):

- Calories: 120
- Protein: 15g
- Carbs: 5g
- Fat: 5g

INGREDIENTS

- 1 (5-ounce) can tuna, drained
- 1 tablespoon plain Greek yogurt
- 1 tablespoon chopped fresh herbs (dill, parsley, chives work well)
- ½ teaspoon lemon juice
- Salt and pepper to taste
- 1-2 cucumbers

DIRECTIONS

1. Combine tuna, Greek yogurt, herbs, lemon juice, salt, and pepper in a bowl.
2. Cut the cucumber(s) in half lengthwise, scoop out some of the seeds to create a little 'boat'.
3. Fill the cucumber boats with the tuna mixture.

Tips

- Add a sprinkle of chopped celery or onion to the tuna mixture for extra crunch.
- For a spicier kick: try a dash of hot sauce or a pinch of red pepper flakes.

Edamame Power

Why We Love It:

- Plant-Based Protein: Edamame packs a vegetarian protein punch.
- Fun to Eat!: Popping those pods is oddly satisfying.
- Fiber Boost: Helps keep you feeling full between meals.

Prep Time: 5 minutes **Cook Time:** Varies depending on the method (5 min steaming, 10-15 roasting)

Approximate Nutritional Info (per ½ cup serving):

- Calories: 100
- Protein: 9g
- Carbs: 8g
- Fat: 4g

INGREDIENTS

- 1 cup frozen shelled edamame
- Sea salt or chili flakes for seasoning

DIRECTIONS

- Steam Option: Steam edamame according to package directions or until tender (about 5 minutes).
- Roast Option: Toss edamame with a tiny bit of olive oil and season. Roast in a preheated 400°F oven for 10-15 minutes, or until slightly browned and crispy.
- Sprinkle with sea salt or chili flakes. Enjoy warm or cold!

Tips

- Buy pre-shelled edamame for convenience.
- Get creative with seasonings: A sprinkle of garlic powder, black pepper, or a squeeze of lemon adds extra flavor.

Spicy Roasted Chickpeas

Why We Love It:

- Crunchy Craving Buster: Satisfies that need for a salty, crunchy snack.
- Full of Flavor: Customizable with your favorite spice combinations.
- Fiber & Protein: The combo keeps you feeling satisfied.

Prep Time: 10 minutes **Cook Time:** 30-40 minutes

Approximate Nutritional Info (per ½ cup serving):

- Calories: 150
- Protein: 7g
- Carbs: 20g
- Fat: 7g

INGREDIENTS

- 1 (15-ounce) can chickpeas, rinsed and drained
- 1 tablespoon olive oil
- 1 teaspoon cumin
- ½ teaspoon paprika
- ¼ teaspoon chili powder
- ¼ teaspoon salt (or to taste)

DIRECTIONS

1. Pat chickpeas dry with a paper towel (this helps them get crispy).
2. Toss chickpeas with olive oil and spices.
3. Roast in a preheated 400°F oven for 30-40 minutes, tossing halfway through, until golden brown and crispy.

Tips

- Adjust spices to your liking: try curry powder, smoked paprika, garlic powder, etc.
- For extra crunch, increase roasting time by 5-10 minutes.
- Store in an airtight container for a few days of snacking.

Turkey Jerky or Beef Strips

Why We Love It:

- Portable Protein: Great for on-the-go or when you need something quick.
- High Protein: Helps curb hunger and supports muscle building. Flavorful: Many brands offer a variety of savory flavors

Prep Time: None! **Cook Time:** None!

Approximate Nutritional Info (per 1 oz serving):

- Calories: 80-100 (can vary depending on brand and flavor)
- Protein: 10-15g
- Carbs: 0-5g (watch for added sugars)
- Fat: 2-4g

INGREDIENTS

- Low-sodium turkey jerky or beef strips

Tips

- Look for brands with simple ingredients and minimal additives.
- Opt for individual servings for better portion control.

DIRECTIONS

1. Read the label carefully! Choose minimally processed jerky with no added sugars.
2. Enjoy as a snack!

Cottage Cheese & Tomato Delight

Why We Love It:
- Creamy & Refreshing: The perfect combo of textures and flavors.
- Protein Power: Cottage cheese is a great source of protein for satiety.
- Easy & Quick: Ready in minutes, perfect for a no-fuss snack.

Prep Time: 5 minutes **Cook Time:** None!

Approximate Nutritional Info (per serving):

- Calories: 150
- Protein: 15g
- Carbs: 10g
- Fat: 5g

INGREDIENTS

- ½ cup cottage cheese
- 1 medium tomato, sliced
- Drizzle of balsamic glaze
- Salt and pepper to taste

DIRECTIONS

1. Top cottage cheese with the sliced tomato.
2. Drizzle with balsamic glaze, season with salt and pepper. Enjoy!

Tips

- Use fresh, ripe tomatoes for the best flavor.
- Add a sprinkle of fresh basil for an extra burst of flavor.
- For a bit of crunch, add chopped cucumbers or a few olives.

Apple & Nut Butter Power

Why We Love It:
- Classic & Satisfying: The sweet and salty combo hits the spot.
- Fiber Filling: Apples provide fiber for sustained energy.
- Healthy Fats: Nut butter delivers good fats and protein.

Prep Time: 5 minutes **Cook Time:** None!

Approximate Nutritional Info (per serving with almond butter):

- Calories: 250
- Protein: 8g
- Carbs: 35g
- Fat: 15g

INGREDIENTS

- 1 apple, sliced
- 2 tablespoons your favorite nut butter (almond, peanut, cashew, etc.)

DIRECTIONS

1. Arrange apple slices on a plate or in a bowl.
2. Serve with nut butter for dipping.

Tips

- Experiment with different apples: Try tart Granny Smith or sweet Honeycrisp.
- Add a sprinkle of cinnamon for an extra boost of flavor.

Cottage Cheese Fruit Salad

Why We Love It:
- Protein & Vitamins Combined: A balanced and nutritious snack.
- Customizable: Swap fruits based on what you have or what's in season.
- Creamy Goodness: Cottage cheese adds a rich and satisfying texture.

Prep Time: 5 minutes **Cook Time:** None!

Approximate Nutritional Info (per serving, without honey):

- Calories: 250
- Protein: 20g
- Carbs: 25g
- Fat: 12g

INGREDIENTS

- ½ cup cottage cheese
- ½ cup mixed berries (blueberries, raspberries, blackberries, strawberries)
- 2 tablespoons chopped nuts (walnuts, almonds, pecans)
- Drizzle of honey (optional)

DIRECTIONS

1. Top cottage cheese with the berries and chopped nuts.
2. Add a drizzle of honey for extra sweetness, if desired.

Tips

- Use any combination of fruits you like: chopped melon, peaches, etc.
- For a tropical twist, try mango and a sprinkle of toasted coconut.

Protein Trail Mix

Why We Love It:
- Energy Booster: Perfect for fueling hikes or a busy day.
- Customizable: Create your perfect flavor combination.
- Portable: Easy to stash in your bag or desk for on-the-go snacking.

Prep Time: 5 minutes **Cook Time:** None!

Approximate Nutritional Info (per ¼ cup serving):

- Calories: 200
- Protein: 8g
- Carbs: 20g
- Fat: 15g

INGREDIENTS

- ¼ cup nuts (almonds, walnuts, cashews, etc.)
- ¼ cup seeds (pumpkin, sunflower, chia)
- ¼ cup unsweetened dried fruit (in moderation - cranberries, raisins, chopped apricots)
- 2 tablespoons dark chocolate chips (optional)

DIRECTIONS

1. Combine all ingredients in a container and enjoy a handful as a snack.

Tips

- Get creative! Add other ingredients like unsweetened coconut flakes or a touch of your favorite spices.
- Control sweetness: adjust the amount of dried fruit and chocolate chips for less sugar.

Yogurt Bark

Why We Love It:
- Creamy & Crunchy: Enjoy the mix of textures from yogurt, toppings, and frozen treats.
- Customizable: Get creative with your favorite flavors and crunchy add-ins.
- Fun to Make: A simple snack that's perfect for getting creative in the kitchen.

Prep Time: 10 minutes + freezing time
Cook Time: None!

Approximate Nutritional Info (per serving):

- Calories: 150
- Protein: 20g
- Carbs: 15g
- Fat: 5g

INGREDIENTS

- 1 cup plain Greek yogurt
- 1 scoop protein powder (vanilla or berry flavor)
- ¼ cup fresh berries (blueberries, raspberries, etc.)
- 2 tablespoons chopped nuts or seeds

DIRECTIONS

1. Mix: Combine Greek yogurt and protein powder until smooth.
2. Spread: Line a baking sheet with parchment paper. Spread the yogurt mixture in a thin layer.
3. Top & Freeze: Sprinkle with berries and chopped nuts (or your favorite toppings). Freeze for at least 2 hours, or until solid.
4. Break & Enjoy: Break into pieces and enjoy as a frozen treat!

Tips

- Experiment with toppings: try granola, unsweetened coconut flakes, a drizzle of melted nut butter, etc.
- For extra sweetness: Add a tiny drizzle of honey or maple syrup to the yogurt mixture before freezing.

Protein Pudding

Why We Love It:

- Decadent & Guilt-Free: Satisfies that sweet tooth without the added sugar.
- Protein Boost: Perfect for a post-workout treat or an afternoon pick-me-up.

Prep Time: 5 minutes **Cook Time:** None!

Approximate Nutritional Info (per serving):

- Calories: 200
- Protein: 30g
- Carbs: 15g
- Fat: 5g

INGREDIENTS

- 1 cup plain Greek yogurt
- 1 scoop protein powder (chocolate or vanilla)
- 2 tablespoons almond milk (or milk of your choice)

DIRECTIONS

1. Mix: Combine Greek yogurt, protein powder, and almond milk. Blend until smooth for a creamier texture.
2. Chill & Enjoy: Refrigerate for a thicker consistency if desired. Enjoy!

Tips

- Top with fresh berries, a sprinkle of nuts, or a few dark chocolate chips for extra flavor.

Protein Roll-Ups

Why We Love It:

- Portable & Delicious: Perfect for a grab-and-go snack or light lunch.
- Customizable: Swap out your favorite nut butter and fruits.
- Balanced Nutrition: A blend of protein, carbs, and healthy fats.

Prep Time: 5 minutes Cook Time: None!

Approximate Nutritional Info (per roll-up):

- **Calories: 280**
- **Protein: 10g**
- **Carbs: 40g**
- **Fat: 13g**

INGREDIENTS

- 1 slice whole-wheat Ezekiel bread
- 2 tablespoons nut butter of your choice
- ½ banana, sliced (or other fruit like berries, sliced apple)
- Sprinkle of cinnamon (optional)

DIRECTIONS

1. Spread: Spread the nut butter evenly onto the Ezekiel bread.
2. Top & Roll: Arrange the banana slices (or other chosen fruit) along one edge of the bread. Sprinkle with cinnamon if desired. Roll tightly.
3. Slice & Enjoy! Slice the roll-up in half for easier eating, if desired.

Tips

- Use sunflower seed butter for a nut-free option.
- Add a drizzle of honey for extra sweetness, but remember this will increase the carb content.

Mini Chicken Salad Cups

Why We Love It:

- Savory Satisfaction: A protein-packed twist on the classic appetizer.
- Easy to Assemble: Perfect for using leftover chicken or grabbing rotisserie chicken.
- Low Carb: Lettuce cups provide a fresh and crunchy base.

Prep Time: 10 minutes
Cook Time: None if using pre-cooked chicken
Approximate Nutritional Info (per 2 lettuce cups):

- **Calories: 120**
- **Protein: 15g**
- **Carbs: 5g**
- **Fat: 5g**

INGREDIENTS

- ½ cup shredded chicken (cooked)
- 2 tablespoons plain Greek yogurt
- 1 tablespoon chopped celery
- Salt and pepper to taste
- 4-6 large lettuce leaves (butter or Boston lettuce work well)

DIRECTIONS

1. Make the Salad: Mix together shredded chicken, Greek yogurt, celery, salt, and pepper.
2. Fill and Enjoy: Spoon chicken salad into the lettuce leaves.

Tips

- Add a sprinkle of your favorite fresh herbs like dill or parsley.
- Get creative with additions: Try chopped grapes, walnuts, or a dash of curry powder.

Savory Protein Muffins

Why We Love It:
- Make-Ahead Meal Prep: Bake a batch on the weekend for easy snacks throughout the week.
- Protein Packed: Perfect for a post-workout snack or a satisfying on-the-go breakfast.
- Flavorful: Loaded with veggies, protein, and satisfying spices.

Prep Time: 10 minutes **Cook Time:** 20-25 minutes

Approximate Nutritional Info (per muffin):

- Calories: 120
- Protein: 10g
- Carbs: 3g
- Fat: 8g

INGREDIENTS

- 6 eggs
- ½ cup chopped spinach
- ¼ cup chopped bell pepper (any color)
- 2 tablespoons crumbled turkey bacon (or cooked sausage)
- ¼ cup shredded cheese
- Salt and pepper to taste

DIRECTIONS

1. Prep & Bake: Preheat oven to 350°F. Grease a muffin tin.
2. Whisk eggs, then stir in spinach, bell pepper, turkey bacon, cheese, salt, and pepper.
3. Divide the mixture evenly among muffin cups. Bake for 20-25 minutes, or until set.

Tips

- Freeze leftovers for easy reheating later.
- Experiment with different veggie and protein combos!

Shrimp Cocktail

Why We Love It:

- Classic & Elegant: Feels like a treat but is low-carb and high in protein.
- Light & Refreshing: Perfect for a warm day or when you want something simple.
- Quick & Easy: Ready in minutes, especially if you buy pre-cooked shrimp.

Prep Time: 5 minutes (if using pre-cooked shrimp) **Cook Time:** None! (if using pre-cooked shrimp)

Approximate Nutritional Info (per serving):

- Calories: 150
- Protein: 25g
- Carbs: 5g
- Fat: 3g

INGREDIENTS

- ½ pound cooked shrimp, peeled and deveined
- Low-sugar cocktail sauce
- Lemon wedges

DIRECTIONS

1. Arrange the shrimp on a serving dish.
2. Serve with cocktail sauce and lemon wedges on the side.

Tips

- Make your own cocktail sauce: Combine ketchup, horseradish, lemon juice, and hot sauce for a healthier option.
- Add other cocktail accompaniments: Try a few slices of avocado, celery sticks, or cherry tomatoes.

Lentil Hummus & Pita Bites

Why We Love It:

- Vegetarian Delight: A filling and flavorful meatless option.
- Fiber & Protein: The combo of lentils and chickpeas keeps you feeling satisfied.
- Make-Ahead Option: The hummus can be prepared in advance.

Prep Time: 15 minutes **Cook Time:** None (if using pre-cooked lentils)

Approximate Nutritional Info (per serving of hummus + pita):

- Calories: 250
- Protein: 10g
- Carbs: 35g
- Fat: 12g

INGREDIENTS

- ½ cup cooked lentils
- ¼ cup tahini
- 2 tablespoons lemon juice
- 1 clove garlic, minced
- 1 tablespoon olive oil
- Salt and pepper to taste
- Whole-wheat pita bread, cut into wedges
- Optional toppings: Sliced cucumber, chopped tomato, olives

DIRECTIONS

1. Make the Hummus: Blend lentils, tahini, lemon juice, garlic, olive oil, salt, and pepper until smooth.
2. Prep & Serve: Warm the pita wedges (toasting is optional). Serve alongside the hummus with optional toppings.

Tips

- Add a sprinkle of paprika or cumin to the hummus for extra flavor.
- Roast your own pita chips. Cut pita into triangles, drizzle with a bit of olive oil, sprinkle with spices, and bake until crispy.

Chia Seed Pudding

Why We Love It:
- Make-Ahead Winner: Prep it the night before for a grab-and-go breakfast or snack.
- Creamy Goodness: Chia seeds create a satisfying pudding-like texture.
- Boosts Fiber: Helps keep you full and supports your digestive health.

Prep Time: 5 minutes + overnight resting **Cook Time:** None!

Approximate Nutritional Info (per serving, without honey):

- Calories: 250
- Protein: 25g
- Carbs: 25g
- Fat: 10g

INGREDIENTS

- ¼ cup chia seeds
- 1 cup milk (almond milk, unsweetened cashew milk, etc.)
- 1 scoop protein powder (vanilla, chocolate, or berry flavor)
- ½ teaspoon honey (optional)
- Toppings: Fresh berries, chopped nuts, etc.

DIRECTIONS

1. Mix & Rest: Combine chia seeds, milk, protein powder, and honey if using. Refrigerate for at least 2 hours, or best overnight.
2. Top & Enjoy: Stir before serving. Top with your favorite berries, chopped nuts, and any other desired

Tips

- Experiment with different flavors: try adding cocoa powder, a sprinkle of cinnamon, or a splash of vanilla extract.

Frozen Yogurt Bites

Why We Love It:
- Refreshing & Healthy: A simple, guilt-free way to satisfy a sweet craving.
- Easy to Make: Requires only two ingredients.
- Fun for Kids: A great way to get kids involved in making healthy snacks.

Prep Time: 10 minutes + freezing time
Cook Time: None!

Approximate Nutritional Info (per 5 yogurt bites):

- Calories: 50
- Protein: 5g
- Carbs: 10g
- Fat: 1g

INGREDIENTS

- 1 cup grapes (red or green)
- 1 cup plain Greek yogurt

Tips

- Experiment with different fruits: Try strawberries, blueberries, or raspberries.
- For extra sweetness: Add a tiny drizzle of honey to the yogurt before dipping.

DIRECTIONS

1. Wash & Dry: Rinse the grapes and pat them thoroughly dry (this helps the yogurt adhere).
2. Dip & Freeze: Dip each grape into the Greek yogurt, coating evenly. Place on a parchment-lined baking sheet. Freeze for at least 2 hours, or until solid.
3. Store & Enjoy: Once frozen, transfer to an airtight container or freezer bag. Enjoy straight from the freezer!

Parmesan Crisps

Why We Love It:
- Savory & Cheesy: Perfect for satisfying that crunchy, salty craving.
- Low-Carb: A delicious way to sneak in a bit of cheese and protein.
- Versatile: Enjoy them plain, dipped in hummus, or used as a base for toppings.

Prep Time: 5 minutes **Cook Time:** 4-6 minutes

Approximate Nutritional Info (per crisp):

- Calories: 50
- Protein: 4g
- Carbs: 1g
- Fat: 4g

INGREDIENTS

- ½ cup grated Parmesan cheese

Tips

- Sprinkle with herbs: Add a pinch of dried oregano, basil, or Italian seasoning before baking.
- After baking: Try topping them with a tiny bit of pesto or tomato sauce for extra flavor.

DIRECTIONS

1. Prep: Preheat oven to 400°F and line a baking sheet with parchment paper.
2. Create Piles: Drop rounded tablespoons of Parmesan cheese onto the baking sheet, leaving a couple of inches between each pile.
3. Bake: Bake for 4-6 minutes, or until golden brown and crisp.
4. Cool & Enjoy: Let them cool completely on the baking sheet before gently lifting them off. Enjoy!

Smoked Salmon Bites

Why We Love It:

- Elegant & Flavorful: A sophisticated snack with a delicious combination of textures.
- High in Omega-3s: Smoked salmon provides healthy fats.
- Protein Boost: Salmon contributes to a satisfying snack.

Prep Time: 10 minutes **Cook Time:** None!

Approximate Nutritional Info (per 2 bites):

- Calories: 100
- Protein: 10g
- Carbs: 5g
- Fat: 5g

INGREDIENTS

- 3-4 ounces smoked salmon, thinly sliced
- ½ cucumber, sliced into rounds
- Greek Yogurt or cream cheese
- Optional: Fresh dill sprigs for garnish

DIRECTIONS

1. Prep the Cucumber: Slice cucumber into bite-sized rounds.
2. Assemble: Top each cucumber round with a small slice of smoked salmon and a dollop of Greek yogurt (or cream cheese).
3. Garnish & Enjoy: Add a tiny sprig of fresh dill for garnish, if desired.

Tips

- Swap the base: Use mini rice cakes instead of cucumbers for a different textural experience.
- Add a squeeze of lemon: A little lemon juice adds a burst of brightness.

Mini Frittatas

Why We Love It:

- Make-Ahead Marvels: Perfect for prepping ahead for busy days.
- Protein Packed: Eggs deliver a satisfying protein boost.
- Customizable: Get creative with your favorite veggie and protein combos.

Prep Time: 10 minutes **Cook Time:** 20-25 minutes

Approximate Nutritional Info (per frittata):

- Calories: 100
- Protein: 10g
- Carbs: 3g
- Fat: 6g

INGREDIENTS

- 6 large eggs
- ¼ cup chopped vegetables (your choice: spinach, mushrooms, bell peppers, etc.)
- 2 tablespoons lean protein (cooked diced chicken, ham, crumbled sausage, etc.)
- ¼ cup shredded cheese
- Salt and pepper to taste

DIRECTIONS

1. Prep & Preheat: Grease a muffin tin. Preheat oven to 350°F.
2. Whisk & Fill: Whisk eggs with salt and pepper. Stir in vegetables, protein, and cheese. Divide evenly among muffin cups.
3. Bake & Enjoy: Bake for 20-25 minutes or until eggs are set. Serve warm or cold.

Tips

- Freeze for later: Make a big batch and freeze leftovers for easy reheating.
- Spice it up: Add a pinch of chili flakes, smoked paprika, or your favorite herbs.

Chapter 8: Beyond the Food

We've spent a lot of time crafting the perfect high-protein, low-calorie, and low-sugar diet. That's the foundation of your weight-loss journey, but it's not the only piece of the puzzle. To maximize your results and optimize your health, we need to broaden our view. This chapter is about unlocking those 'hidden' factors: hydration, exercise, and sleep. They might seem unrelated to food, but trust me – they'll make all the difference!

The Importance of Hydration: How Much to Drink and Why It Matters

Let's face it, plain water can get boring. But before you reach for sugary drinks, remember this: your body often mistakes thirst for hunger. Staying properly hydrated is one of the easiest ways to curb cravings and support a healthy metabolism.

1. **Aim High:** So, how much water is enough? A good starting point is half your body weight in ounces. So, if you weigh 160 pounds, shoot for 80 ounces (about ten 8oz glasses) of water per day.

2. **Spice Things Up:** If plain water is a struggle, infuse it! Add slices of lemon, cucumber, berries, or mint for a refreshing twist. Unsweetened herbal teas count towards your fluid intake too.

3. **Listen to Your Body:** Check your urine color – a pale yellow means you're on track. Darker yellow indicates you need to up your water game.

Why Hydration is Key, Especially on This Plan:

- **Protein Needs Water:** Your body uses water to process protein efficiently. Dehydration can hinder this, making you feel sluggish and bloated.
- **Goodbye Fake Hunger:** Being well-hydrated helps differentiate true hunger from thirst signals, preventing unnecessary snacking.
- **Waste Not, Want Not:** Proper hydration helps your body flush out toxins and waste products, essential for optimal health and energy levels.

Exercise Basics: Integrating Movement into Your Weight Loss Journey

Let's be honest, exercise can feel like a chore. But what if we reframed it as a superpower, not an obligation? Here's why movement matters!

1. **Calorie Torch:** Sure, diet is primary for weight loss, but exercise burns extra calories, boosting your results significantly.

2. **Muscle = Metabolism:** Muscle tissue burns more calories at rest than fat tissue. Strength training helps you build that metabolism-boosting muscle.

3. **Beyond the Scale:** Exercise improves body composition, meaning you might see inches lost and clothes fitting better, even if the scale doesn't budge much initially.

Getting Started, Your Way:

- **Find Your Fun:** If you hate running, don't do it! Explore dancing, swimming, hiking, or team sports. Movement should be joyful as often as possible.

- **Small Steps, Big Wins:** Start with 10-15 minutes a few days a week. Consistency is more important than intensity, especially at the beginning.

- **Strength Counts:** Don't underestimate bodyweight exercises: Squats, lunges, push-ups – these build muscle and can be done anywhere!

Sleep for Success: Emphasize Sleep's Role in Metabolism and Hunger

Sleep is the ultimate reset button, yet it's often the first thing we sacrifice. Bad news: skimping on sleep seriously sabotages your weight loss efforts.

1. **Hanger Monster:** Sleep deprivation ramps up hunger hormones and makes you crave sugary, high-carb foods for quick energy.

2. **Metabolism Blues:** Not getting enough sleep disrupts your body's natural rhythm, potentially slowing down your metabolism.

3. **Stress City:** Lack of sleep increases the stress hormone cortisol, which encourages fat storage, especially around your belly.

The Sleep Sweet Spot:

- **7-8 Hours is Ideal:** Most adults need this much for optimal function.
- **Consistency is Queen:** Try to stick to a regular sleep schedule, even on weekends.
- **Power Down:** Create a relaxing bedtime routine: dim lights, turn off electronics, take a warm bath.

Remember, it's about Progress, Not Perfection. Don't get overwhelmed – even small changes in hydration, movement, and sleep stack up over time. Celebrate your wins, no matter how small, and keep building those healthy habits!

Chapter 9: The Power of Planning – Your 12-Week Blueprint

The last few chapters armed you with all the delicious recipes and nutritional know-how. Now, we're layering in strategy. A well-crafted meal plan is like a roadmap. It removes guesswork, reduces impulsive choices, and streamlines your success!

Your Meal Planning Toolkit:

The Planner:

- ➤ **Meals:** Breakfast, lunch, dinner, and snacks for each day of the week.
- ➤ **Grocery List:** Organized to match your plan, making shopping a breeze.
- ➤ **Nutrition Tracker:** Spaces to jot down your calorie and protein goals, and a running tally for each day.

Recipe Bank: Those recipes we've explored? They're your building blocks! Choose ones that fit your taste and your high-protein, low-carb, low-sugar parameters.

Goal Awareness: Keep your daily calorie and protein targets in mind as you build your plan. A calculator or food-tracking app comes in handy here.

<u>Let's Build: Using a Sample Week</u>

Day	Meal 1	Meal 2	Meal 3	Meal 4	Meal 5	Total Calories	Total Protein
Day 1	Protein Oatmeal (mod. recipe) + Berries	Greek Yogurt Dip & Veggies(pg.58)	Half Portion Tuna Cucumber Boats (3-4 Boats) + Salad(pg60)	Savory Protein Muffin (1) + Small Greek Yogurt (pg. 72)	Lemon Garlic Salmon (pg. 46) (small portion) + Asparagus	1300-1500	105g
Day 2	Greek Yogurt w/ protein powder, berries, sprinkle of nuts(pg.58)	Lentil & Egg Super Salad (half portion) + crackers(pg.30)	Mini Chicken Salad Cups (3-4 cups) (pg. 71)	Apple with Nut Butter + Hard-boiled Egg (pg. 65)	Spicy Peanut Chicken Stir-fry (less sauce, extra veggies, moderate portion) (pg. 43)	1200-1600	100-120g
Day 3	Cottage Cheese Fruit Salad (moderate portion) (pg. 66)	Savory Protein Muffin (1) + hummus (pg. 72)	Greek Shrimp & Feta Salad (light dressing) (pg. 31)	Shrimp Cocktail (4-5) + veggies (pg. 73)	Tofu & Veggie Power Bowl (mod. portion) (pg. 49)	1200-1600	100-120g
Day 4	Eggs in Purgatory (2 eggs, lean protein) (pg. 56)	Tuna Cucumber Boats (3-4) + Salad (pg. 60)	Lentil & Spinach Curry (mod. portion) over cauliflower rice (pg. 51)	Protein Trail Mix (handful) + Greek yogurt (pg.67)	Black Bean Veggie Wrap (small tortilla/lettuce wrap) (pg. 34)	1200-1600	100-120g
Day 5	Protein Pudding (small) + berries (pg. 69)	Spicy Lentil & Chicken Soup (small portion) + salad (pg. 35)	Smoked Salmon Bites (3-4) + salad (pg. 78)	Edamame + Cottage Cheese (pg. 61& 66)	Mini Frittatas (2) with side salad (pg. 79)	1200-1600	100-120g
Day 6	2 Egg White & Veggie Scramble (pg. 23)	Protein Roll-Up (1) + veggies (pg. 70)	Chicken Quinoa Fiesta (mod. portion) (pg. 29)	Greek Yogurt Dip & Veggies(pg.58) + Spicy Roasted Chickpeas(pg.62)	Turkey Meatballs (mod. portion) with Zucchini Noodles & light marinara (pg. 54)	1200-1600	100-120g
Day 7	Protein Oatmeal (mod. portion) + Berries	Cottage Cheese & Tomato Delight + crackers (pg. 64)	Tuna Steak Power Bowl (emphasis on tuna) (pg. 47)	Hard-boiled Egg with crackers (pg. 59)	Shrimp Scampi (small portion) with Zucchini Noodles (pg.48)	1200-1600	100-120g

Repeat & Adapt: You'd follow this process for each day of the week, choosing different recipes, always aiming to hit your calorie and protein goals.

Variety is Key: Avoid repetition – it leads to boredom and burnout. Mix in different recipes to keep meals exciting.

Prep Power: Set aside a time for batch cooking or meal prep on weekends. This saves HUGE time during busy weekdays.

Flexibility: Plans are GUIDES, not prison sentences. If a recipe doesn't work on a particular day, swap it out!

The Magic: Why Meal Planning Works

- **Control:** You dictate what goes into your body, avoiding last-minute unhealthy choices.
- **Mindfulness:** The tracking keeps you aware of your intake.
- **Efficiency:** Less time spent wondering "what's for dinner?" means more time for the things you love.

Chapter 10: Transitioning to Maintenance

You've put in the hard work for those 12 weeks, diligently followed your high-protein, low-calorie, low-sugar plan, and you've seen fantastic results! But what comes next? This chapter is your guide to navigating the shift from active weight loss to a sustainable, healthy lifestyle that will keep those results long after the initial goal is achieved.

Life after the 12 Weeks: Gradually Increase Carbs & Calories

1. **Slow & Steady Wins the Race:** The danger in ending a diet is the sudden, drastic shift back to old habits. It's tempting, but this often leads to rapid weight regain. Instead, we'll gradually reintroduce more carbs and calories to find your maintenance level.

2. **Carb Cycling:** Start by adding healthy carbs (think whole grains, sweet potato, fruits) on 1-2 days of the week. Observe how your body responds – how's your energy, hunger, and weight? If all goes well, add another carb day.

3. **Calorie Bump:** Simultaneously, slightly increase your daily calories by 100-200. Focus on adding healthy fats (avocado, nuts, olive oil) and lean protein. Continue tracking your intake.

4. **Listen to Your Body:** Are you still losing weight? Increase a bit more. Feeling a bit sluggish? Scale back slightly. This is a process of finding your body's sweet spot.

Making It Sustainable: Creating a Healthy, Balanced Lifestyle Long-Term

Weight maintenance is NOT about deprivation. It's about finding a way of eating and living that feels good, sustainable, and allows you to enjoy life.

- ✓ **The 80/20 Rule:** Strive for 80% of your meals to be those nutrient-dense, healthy choices you've learned. The other 20%? Give yourself guilt-free space to enjoy occasional treats - birthdays, dinners out, etc.

- ✓ **Ditch the Diet Mentality:** This isn't temporary - it's a lifestyle shift. Release the all-or-nothing thinking, allowing for flexibility and moderation.

- ✓ **Focus on Habits:** What habits helped you succeed during those first 12 weeks? Meal planning? Prioritizing protein? Identify the non-negotiables and keep them in your routine.

- ✓ **Find Your Joy (Beyond Food):** What else nourishes you besides food? Movement you enjoy? Time outdoors? Social connection? Invest in those areas – they are also vital for long-term health.

- ✓ **Stay Mindful:** Continue self-monitoring. Regularly checking in with your body - weight, energy levels, how clothes fit - keeps you aware of any creeping shifts.

Bonus Section

Meal Planner

Week 1	Meal 1	Meal 2	Meal 3	Meal 4	Meal 5	Total Calories	Total Protein
Day 1							
Day 2							
Day 3							
Day 4							
Day 5							
Day 6							
Day 7							

Week 2	Meal 1	Meal 2	Meal 3	Meal 4	Meal 5	Total Calories	Total Protein
Day 1							
Day 2							
Day 3							
Day 4							
Day 5							
Day 6							
Day 7							

Week 3	Meal 1	Meal 2	Meal 3	Meal 4	Meal 5	Total Calories	Total Protein
Day 1							
Day 2							
Day 3							
Day 4							
Day 5							
Day 6							
Day 7							

Week 4	Meal 1	Meal 2	Meal 3	Meal 4	Meal 5	Total Calories	Total Protein
Day 1							
Day 2							
Day 3							
Day 4							
Day 5							
Day 6							
Day 7							

Week 5	Meal 1	Meal 2	Meal 3	Meal 4	Meal 5	Total Calories	Total Protein
Day 1							
Day 2							
Day 3							
Day 4							
Day 5							
Day 6							
Day 7							

Week 6	Meal 1	Meal 2	Meal 3	Meal 4	Meal 5	Total Calories	Total Protein
Day 1							
Day 2							
Day 3							
Day 4							
Day 5							
Day 6							
Day 7							

Week 7	Meal 1	Meal 2	Meal 3	Meal 4	Meal 5	Total Calories	Total Protein
Day 1							
Day 2							
Day 3							
Day 4							
Day 5							
Day 6							
Day 7							

Week 8	Meal 1	Meal 2	Meal 3	Meal 4	Meal 5	Total Calories	Total Protein
Day 1							
Day 2							
Day 3							
Day 4							
Day 5							
Day 6							
Day 7							

Week 9	Meal 1	Meal 2	Meal 3	Meal 4	Meal 5	Total Calories	Total Protein
Day 1							
Day 2							
Day 3							
Day 4							
Day 5							
Day 6							
Day 7							

Week 10	Meal 1	Meal 2	Meal 3	Meal 4	Meal 5	Total Calories	Total Protein
Day 1							
Day 2							
Day 3							
Day 4							
Day 5							
Day 6							
Day 7							

Week 11	Meal 1	Meal 2	Meal 3	Meal 4	Meal 5	Total Calories	Total Protein
Day 1							
Day 2							
Day 3							
Day 4							
Day 5							
Day 6							
Day 7							

Week 12	Meal 1	Meal 2	Meal 3	Meal 4	Meal 5	Total Calories	Total Protein
Day 1							
Day 2							
Day 3							
Day 4							
Day 5							
Day 6							
Day 7